Getting High

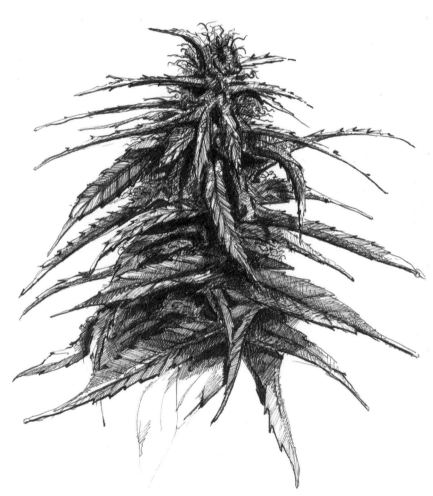

Mature female flowering top.

Getting High

Marijuana through the Ages

John Charles Chasteen

ROWMAN & LITTLEFIELD
Lanham • Boulder • New York • London

Published by Rowman & Littlefield
A wholly owned subsidiary of The Rowman & Littlefield Publishing Group, Inc.
4501 Forbes Boulevard, Suite 200, Lanham, Maryland 20706
www.rowman.com

Unit A, Whitacre Mews, 26-34 Stannary Street, London SE11 4AB, United
Kingdom

Distributed by NATIONAL BOOK NETWORK

British Library Cataloguing in Publication Information Available

Library of Congress Cataloging-in-Publication Data
Chasteen, John Charles, 1955– author.
  Getting high : marijuana through the ages / John Charles Chasteen.
    pages cm
  Includes bibliographical references and index.
  ISBN 978-1-4422-5469-5 (cloth : alk. paper) — ISBN 978-1-4422-5470-1
(electronic) 1. Marijuana abuse—History. 2. Marijuana—History. I. Title.
  HV5822.M3C43 2016
  362.29'509—dc23

                                                        2015027167

Printed in the United States of America

To the Riamba Bros.
actual and honorary
living and dead

Contents

1

❋

Getting High

Just wait until people our age are running things. Then everything will change. My sixteen-year-old friends and I had no doubts in the matter, around 1970. We assured each other, when we smoked marijuana, that a new dawn was inevitable in a world that was "turning on." Marijuana, we believed, was a "mind-expanding" drug, somewhat like LSD, but much milder. The distinction was blurred, anyway, because we often used them together. We supposed that anyone, particularly anyone young, would change their attitude, spontaneously abandoning racism or support of the Vietnam War, for example, under the mind-expanding influence of the drug. Marijuana would help anyone see through sham and resist mind control by "The System." The problem was getting them off booze, which dulled perceptions, rather than heightening them.

My sixteen-year-old friends and I viewed getting high and getting drunk as rough opposites. Marijuana was the drug of our tribe, the cool, long-haired, rock-music-listening, faded-blue-jean-wearing tribe. Pot, as we called it most often, made people peaceful. Alcohol belonged to the *other* tribe, exemplified by hard-hat construction workers who drank beer and threatened to beat up "long-hairs." Alcohol stood for decadent tradition, and it made people violent.

We were wrong, of course, about the world, and also about pot's irresistible persuasiveness. The world proved harder to remake than we had ever supposed. And the clarity of the 1970 tribes soon got muddled. By the 1990s, when I was a college professor sipping wine at faculty parties, men with long hair seemed more likely to be construction workers than students. Pot and beer no longer seemed like opposites, either. Marijuana's mind-expanding qualities had gotten lost.

Did it ever really possess them?

This book looks at marijuana in the long view of world history. It asks who used it, how, and why. Unlike most published versions of the drug's history, it places marijuana within larger historical patterns, such as migration, colonialism, and religion. It also keeps the marijuana/beer comparison in mind throughout. Above all, it asks whether marijuana really possesses mind-expanding powers.

A simple question, perhaps, but without a simple answer. For starters, the effects of the drug are variable and subjective. Consider the complexities. The same dose can affect different people differently, and the same person differently at different moments. That's true of alcohol, too, but truer of marijuana. Its effect will vary according to expectations. To a degree, altered consciousness is always a blank screen onto which people project their expectations. Expectations play an enormous role in people's reaction to *any* drug, of course, which is why placebos work. All this plays havoc with our attempts to characterize marijuana's mind-altering qualities in the abstract.

To understand the effects of mind-altering drugs, it's better to ask how they are *used* in everyday life. Like alcohol, marijuana is often used just for fun. That is because, like alcohol, it is a "euphoriant" that triggers a surge of dopamine in the brains of users. Many recreational drugs are euphoriants, but their effects vary. The point of recreational use is simply to enhance the moment by stepping out of ordinary consciousness. Often, the fact that drugs *somehow* alter ordinary consciousness matters more than just *how* they alter it. Recreational use is generally social. It facilitates interpersonal bonding and generally greases the social gears. That is why, like drinking alcohol, smoking marijuana is very commonly a collective activity. In the late-twentieth-century United States, millions of people who smoked marijuana socially when they were university students, drank alcohol socially later in life, getting fundamentally the same thing out of it, a shared experience of release from the ordinary.

Still, the two drugs contrast in some respects. Alcohol depresses the nervous system; marijuana does not. At high doses, the drinker may experience difficulty walking or, famously, pronouncing words, and may black out or even, in extreme cases, die. Marijuana does not have those effects even at high doses. Instead, it creates distortions of normal perception and thought, as well as measurable deficits in reaction time, cognition, concentration, and memory. At high doses, it can produce visual hallucinations, such as the strobing arm movements that made my teenage friends look a little like Hindu deities. This is why pharmacologists tend to classify alcohol as a depressant, whereas they call marijuana's cognitive effects "hallucinogenic." The hallucinogenic effects, not shared by alcohol, seem to explain marijuana's allegedly mind-expanding qualities.

Scientific research now demonstrates that marijuana is a medical drug, too. A hundred years ago we knew that, but we'd forgotten. Cannabis has always figured in the pharmacopoeias of Europe and China, although these traditional medical uses, such as hempseed oil in the ear for earache, or cannabis-leaf poultices on a sprain, did not involve getting high. In addition, the euphoriant effect, when present, is a palliative that makes any ill more bearable. In the twenty-first century, research has revealed further medical uses. Marijuana's unique active ingredients, called *cannabinoids* (THC is the best known), have molecular shapes that fit receptors in our body's hormonal communication systems, regulating mood and appetite, among other things. That's how marijuana can calm chronic seizures or restore appetite and reduce pain and nausea in patients undergoing chemotherapy or enduring AIDS, for example. At least one therapeutic cannabinoid molecule, called CBD, is not mood-altering at all. Moreover, cannabinoids have few deleterious side effects. There are pharmaceutical imitations, but the synthetics do not seem to provide the same kind of relief.

Because experiments with cannabinoids led to the discovery of the hormonal system they affect, researchers call it the "endocannabinoid system." Note that this choice of name does *not* demonstrate that the human hormonal system evolved in conjunction with marijuana, however, as some have fantasized.

Ideas about the effects of marijuana have undergone several dramatic shifts in recent history. In the 1930s—which is *very* recent history on the global scale—marijuana was condemned by the U.S. government and the mass media as a "devil weed" that drove users criminally and violently insane. My teenage friends and I flocked (high, of course) to see midnight showings of the 1930s propaganda movie *Reefer Madness*, which by the 1970s seemed ridiculous to pretty much everybody. The 1970s audience died laughing, but the movie makers had been deadly serious. After all, Harry Anslinger, the head of the Federal Bureau of Narcotics, had secured passage of the 1937 federal law making marijuana illegal partly by showing photographs of bloodied corpses—the typical work, he indicated, of the "reefer mad." He also deployed historical evidence, so to speak, claiming that the English word *assassin* derives, ultimately, from a sort of reefer madness that had existed in medieval Syria. We'll take a closer look at that idea later in the book. For now, let's note how absolutely the "assassin" image contrasted with that of pot-smoking hippies preaching "peace and love" in the 1960s. Then, by the 1980s and 1990s, another contrasting image emerged. Now the stereotypical marijuana smokers became stoner "couch potatoes," antisocial and riddled with "amotivational syndrome."

This variability is mostly a matter of social expectations, no doubt, but pharmacology helps explain it somewhat. THC, short for delta-9-tetrahydrocannabinol, is apparently the most mind-altering cannabinoid, but there are more than fifty others, at least three of which are also psychoactive. Different strains of cannabis—even, to a degree, individual plants—have differing endowments of cannabinoids. Furthermore, they interact, so their differing endowments create kaleidoscopic variations. (In contrast, a single molecule, *ethanol*, is the sole active ingredient of all alcoholic drinks.) Today's cannabis connoisseurs, focusing on various strains sold as medical marijuana, say that more *sativa* hybrids go to the head, make one "high" without impeding activity, while more *indica* hybrids register in the body, making one more "stoned" and lethargic. Whatever . . .

Here's the point. Marijuana is a mind-expanding drug when (and only when) people learn to use it that way. My teenage cronies and I did not invent such effects, nor did we discover them for ourselves. Instead, we read about them in books and magazines, heard about them on television and in the lyrics of rock music, before we ever tried marijuana. Perhaps the most influential description of the drug came from the poet Allen Ginsberg in his famous 1966 *Atlantic Monthly* article "The Great Marijuana Hoax," which he wrote partly high and partly not in order to demonstrate marijuana's effects on his thinking. His overall idea was that marijuana stimulates unconventional, and therefore creative, thought, which is what makes it interesting to artists. It was an idea famously shared by Jamaican reggae musicians, who believed that *ganja*, as they called marijuana, opened their minds to divine inspiration. Nor did Ginsberg and his generation make up this idea, of course. Early jazz players, such as Louis Armstrong, had their own version of it, as we will see. And so, too, did untold generations of ascetic holy men of Central and Southwest Asia, Sufis and Sannyasins who renounced the world in their spiritual quest.

In fact, when one looks at who's been using cannabis drugs in the last two or three thousand years, one sees that they have been mostly spiritual, rather than recreational, users. In other words, the drug has been prized more as a hallucinogen than a euphoriant. Cannabis use as a recreational euphoriant has, in fact, been rare in global history, concentrated in a few societies, never rivaling the social importance of alcohol. Recreational use of marijuana is rather modern, occurring most widely during the last century, whereas the spiritual uses are much older. In sum, the big picture of world history suggests that human beings have used marijuana *most often* as a mind-expanding drug.

TROUBLE WITH THE POLICE

Why, then, is marijuana illegal? That's the first question that any reasonable person is likely to ask at this point, and it deserves a straight answer. How did this very ancient and widespread crop, one of humankind's original domesticated plants, become banned more or less worldwide? The gist of the answer lies in the next chapter.

For now, contemplate the dramatic impact of today's anti-marijuana laws. The drug's general illegality is among the first things anyone learns about it. In my case, as a middle-class American kid, I learned it from the 1960s televised detective series *Dragnet*, and then from the local broadcast news report, which ominously showed the house of family friends as a crime scene. Marijuana's illegality constitutes a major reason why the United States now keeps more of its population in prison, by far, than other countries. Roughly half of the drug offenses tabulated annually by the FBI involve marijuana, and roughly half the inmates in federal penitentiaries are there for selling or, sometimes, for merely possessing it. The rampant incarceration associated with the "drug war" has weighed particularly on minority communities in the United States. Some police departments in the United States have begun routinely to seize the property of people accused of possessing marijuana, and they often keep the property without filing formal charges. In essence, it's an institutionalized form of bribery and police corruption: "You had marijuana in your car, so we'll keep both marijuana and car, and you'll say nothing or face drug charges." The main evidence of criminal activity landing many young New Yorkers in jail, when they are profiled and then "stopped and frisked," is a small amount of marijuana. The pervasive drug-testing programs maintained by many businesses effectively target only marijuana, which is detectable in the blood for a month, whereas the traces of other drugs disappear after a few days.

Since the 1970s, U.S. federal law has retained marijuana on its list of most-prohibited "controlled substances," those that it is a crime merely to possess and cannot be consumed under any circumstances. Despite advances in scientific understanding of the body's endocannabinoid system, federal law still specifies that marijuana has "no currently accepted medical use." This is the wording of the Controlled Substances Act, which lists marijuana in its "most dangerous" category, Schedule I, reserved for drugs that also produce "potentially severe psychological or physical dependence." Meanwhile, state laws have begun to vary, beginning with California's Compassionate Use Act of 1996, the first to permit possession and use of marijuana by a doctor's prescription.

The Compassionate Use Act emerged quite specifically in the wake of California's AIDS epidemic. About a dozen mostly western states followed suit in the early 2000s. By 2014, four western states—Washington, Oregon, Colorado, and Alaska—had legalized recreational use of the drug. The advent of the twenty-first century seemed to mark a turning point in the country's approach to marijuana.

Still, state initiatives to license and tax marijuana dispensaries are creating tension with the federal Drug Enforcement Administration, which refuses to recognize the dispensaries' state and local licenses. Diverse observers have noticed that some of the young men buying medical marijuana do not seem very sick. Moreover, serious considerations arise from the problem of producing legal marijuana for legal consumers. Various state laws have made provision for medical marijuana patients to grow a small number of plants for themselves. Mostly, however, the supply comes from licensed dispensaries, which buy marijuana from farmers (or indoor horticulturalists) whose activities are sometimes licensed and sometimes not. Decriminalization and legalization clearly stimulate demand, and demand stimulates supply.

Supplying the demand created by millions of U.S. marijuana consumers—recreational and medical—has become a multimillion-dollar business. The demand is being met mostly by domestic production, both indoors and outdoors, in many states, especially western ones. Related growth is occurring north of the Canadian border in British Columbia. U.S. "homegrown" was once the worst-quality marijuana, but since the 1980s, domestic growers have crossed and selectively bred varieties of marijuana to an unprecedented degree, making U.S. (and Canadian) pot the most potent (and costly) anywhere. At many hundreds of dollars an ounce, its new price constitutes a radical departure from historical patterns. Many players, including some major corporations, are eyeing the market.

Until the drug war, marijuana had always been inexpensive when compared with, say, beer. Now, thanks to vigorous efforts to eradicate the burgeoning domestic crop and interdict illegal importation, high-grade marijuana retails for many dollars a gram. The vast resulting profits have attracted ruthless criminal organizations capable of building their own telecommunications networks and digging freight tunnels under the border between Tijuana and San Diego. Prohibition of marijuana has become a bonanza for organized crime, precisely as occurred in the 1920s with the prohibition of alcohol, except that these new mafias operate internationally. Various criminal trade cartels originating in Jamaica, Colombia, Venezuela, and, more recently, Mexico and Central America have become powerful enough to threaten the integrity of these countries' governments. Turf wars among criminal traffickers produce horrific bloodshed. In recent years, the violence has been most intense in Mexico and Central America, as various militarized criminal syndicates vie with one another to supply the U.S. market. The U.S. market is their major market, too. The level of consumption in Mexico—as measured by "annual prevalence," the proportion of the population that uses it at least once a year—is about a tenth of the U.S. level, according the UN *World Drug Report*.

Increasingly, state-level legalization makes the mayhem of the drug war look irrational. While attitudes have fluctuated since the 1960s, reliable opinion surveys have found that by 2013 a growing majority of Americans, especially the young, believed that marijuana should be legalized. A substantial older, more rural, and more religious minority remains quite opposed, however, and "rescheduling" marijuana at the federal level seems unlikely in an era of Republican political hegemony. State-level initiatives have been notably rare in culturally conservative southern and midwestern states. The West, instead, with its countercultural and also libertarian traditions, has led the way. Medical marijuana initiatives and subsequent legalization of recreational use did not emerge from a cultural vacuum. For example, the author of California's landmark 1996 medical marijuana law, Dennis Peron, was a San Francisco gay-rights activist whose dying partner had been incarcerated for use of marijuana. To judge by the rapid multiplication of licensed dispensaries, smoking marijuana was already pretty common in the communities where they have opened.

Despite changing attitudes, we may well see an enduring split between red states and blue and a standoff at the federal level. Forty years ago, the National Commission on Marihuana and Drug Abuse reached the conclusion that, when it came to its status in the United States, the drug's main sins were essentially political. It's still true. The Shafer Commission, so called for its Republican chairman, named by President Nixon, was the federal government's most notable attempt ever to decide the legal status of marijuana by thoughtful study. This panel of medical experts found occasional recreational use of marijuana to be relatively safe, although it *was* concerned about the much smaller number of daily users. Its members worried, too, that marijuana might lead to experimentation with "harder" drugs, particularly heroin. The commissioners found in marijuana use no social harms, in other words, to rank with alcoholism. At the end of their deliberations, however, wavering between decriminalization and outright legalization, they bowed to public opinion. According to their survey data, in the early 1970s an ample majority of Americans viewed marijuana as simply wrong and "a rejection of enduring American values." That decided the commissioners against legalization. Instead, the Shafer commission recommended the *decriminalization* of marijuana use, whereby people would not be prosecuted for using or possessing small quantities, while commercialization would remain criminal, as had been the case with alcohol in the 1920s.

But the commission's recommendation fell on deaf ears. Faced with a conflict between science and the instincts of his political base, the president who had appointed the Shafer Commission simply ignored its findings. By that time, he had already preemptively declared a "War on Drugs."

Meanwhile, the old idea of "reefer madness" has been definitively discarded, along with the old idea of marijuana's addictiveness. This was a big change from the early twentieth century, when marijuana was called a "narcotic," a loose category that then included cocaine, too. The idea of addiction was then popularly associated with all "narcotics." The real narcotics—opium and its "opiate" derivatives morphine and heroin, as well as synthetic "opioids"—truly are addictive. They produce physical withdrawal symptoms when suddenly discontinued, "cold turkey." Since the 1960s, researchers have recognized that marijuana does not create that kind of "physical addiction."

Some still suggest that marijuana can nonetheless be habit-forming, and they are surely correct. To satisfy any kind of craving can be habit-forming. There need not be any drug involved. Recent experimental science is able to see habits forming at the molecular level, so to speak. It turns out that our brain's response to euphoriant drugs resembles our brain's response to substances like "comfort foods" and activities like gambling and sex. Habitual stimulation of the brain's "pleasure circuit" centers over time "hardwires" neurological circuitry toward the source of stimulation. Simultaneously, though, it also buffers neuronal transmissions at the synapses, thereby encouraging similar—and more intense—stimulation. What was once called "psychological dependence" can now be understood as a neurological process by which people become oriented toward a particular source of pleasure, be it marijuana or alcohol, tobacco or pornography, roulette or bacon.

Given current scientific knowledge, federal prohibition of marijuana lacks any logical basis. Federal scheduling incorrectly declares the drug to have no medical applications. Alcohol and tobacco both present greater health risks. The most persuasive arguments against legalizing marijuana focus on children, because of their evident greater vulnerability than adults. Psychologists have described juvenile amotivational syndrome, a socially isolating, long-term dependence that leads to apathy, bad grades, poor choice of friends, and emotional alienation from parents. Amotivational syndrome figures prominently in parent-centered campaigns against drug abuse. Another discredited but persistently evoked threat to children is that of the hypothetical "gateway drug," admitted to be more or less harmless in itself but threatening because it leads to "harder" drugs, such as heroin.

Clearly, drugs in general are bad for children, but the idea that marijuana inherently threatens them more than alcohol or tobacco is just fear-mongering. An illegal gateway drug is more easily sampled by young people, because buying illegal drugs requires no age identification. Illegality itself constitutes the gateway to be entered. Once inside the gate, one grows used to breaking the law and encounters various other drugs in the illegal marketplace. Take away the illegality, and the gateway disappears. Amotivational syndrome and the gateway-drug idea are effective anti-marijuana arguments, not because they are strong arguments, but because they are about protecting the young, an area where we want to err on the side of caution. They are really not specifically about the effects of marijuana. In fact, a hundred years ago, protecting the young was a principal argument for the prohibition of alcohol.

Which brings us to the last-ditch argument against marijuana. This argument begins by admitting marijuana to be no worse than alcohol and by recognizing the failed experience of national Prohibition in the 1920s. Nonetheless, continues this line of argumentation, we should strive to feel "high on life" without any chemical "crutch." Legalizing other recreational drugs will "send the wrong message" to young people because—and here's the nub—euphoriant drugs are bad. They distract people from the path to true happiness. We should strive for a "drug-free society." Whether or not it mentions religion, this argument is based on moral values derived from religious faith. Many Christians, Muslims, and even Buddhists share this idea. Reasonable people can disagree, but this attitude of moral censure is politically potent, especially in the United States. It's rather reminiscent, in my view, of the sentiment that persuaded the Shafer Commission not to recommend legalization of marijuana in the 1970s.

A final impact of marijuana's current illegality has more practical than moral ramifications. Not all cannabis is marijuana. The distinctive five-pointed compound leaf so well known in the United States as marijuana also belongs to common *hemp*, which does not possess enough cannabinoids to get anyone high. The currently accepted scientific name of both marijuana and hemp is *Cannabis sativa*. The men who wrote the 1937 law making marijuana effectively illegal did not differentiate it from hemp. They defined "marihuana" as "all parts of the plant *Cannabis sativa*." The result was to abolish the well-established U.S. hemp crop overnight, except for a brief federal program that encouraged growing "Hemp for Victory" during World War II. Today, processed hemp fiber and hempseed oil can be imported from Canada and several European countries, as can sterilized hempseed for bird food, but hemp itself can still not be grown in the United States. Proponents of hemp legalization have good (although frequently overblown) arguments to make in favor of the crop, which has many applications. The arguments against legalizing it still cite the difficulty of telling hemp and marijuana apart. What, exactly, is the difference? To trace marijuana's progress around the world, we will have to know it when we see it.

MEET THE CANNABIS PLANT

Hemp was wrongfully incriminated in 1937, so to speak, by its close botanical relationship to marijuana. The hemp form of cannabis had been a common crop in Europe, and then in the United States, for centuries. Never, before the 1900s, however, did it occur to anyone that a drug could be derived from domestic European hemp. To see why, you have to watch the plant grow.

Plant cannabis seeds close together, and the seedlings race upward toward the sunlight in competition with each other, becoming mostly stem. A hemp crop looks a little like a field of skinny, tangled, impossibly dense, ten-foot-tall bamboo. Hemp farmers grow their crop for the long, cane-like stem, because that's where the fibers are. Plant cannabis seeds far apart, on the other hand, and the result is less stemmy, much shorter, more like a bush, with denser foliage and more developed flowers. Marijuana farmers grow their crop for the flowers, especially, because that's where the cannabinoids are concentrated. Almost no one smokes cannabis leaves, particularly no one with access to the flowers.

A further complication: only female flowers will do. Unlike most plants, which have pistils and stamens in the same flower, cannabis has them in separate flowers and, almost always, on separate plants. Pollen tumbles out of tiny, pale yellow, bell-shaped male flowers and is carried by the wind to the female flowers, which are hard to recognize as such. Wind-pollinated plants don't have to attract insects with nectar or colored flower petals. The female cannabis flower is a greenish cluster of slender, feathery, translucent tendrils, called stigmas, which reach out a few millimeters hoping that floating pollen will come to rest on them. On and around the clusters of stigmas the blooming plant exudes a resin rich in cannabinoids.

If the flowers are pollinated, they stop blooming, produce no more resin, and go to seed. To grow a crop of abundantly blooming female plants, marijuana farmers cull male plants. In the males' absence, the never-to-be-pollinated female plants gamely persevere, producing more and more groping tendrils and more sticky resin, until finally they give up the ghost, leaving, at the end of each branch, a dense and withered clump of rust-colored stigmas and resinous crystals without seeds, a *sin semilla* bud. The clusters of sin semilla buds at the top of a single large plant can retail today in the United States for many thousands of dollars.

Marijuana and hemp are above all *crops*, products of cultivation. A cannabis plant only produces sin semilla (and all medical-grade marijuana is sin semilla) if the males are culled, as we have seen. Hemp farmers, on the other hand, grow both male and female plants. They harvest most of the crop *before* it flowers, because flowering takes the plant's energies and degrades the fiber. They do allow a portion of the crop to flower and make seeds for next year's crop. As wind-born hemp pollen blows through the thicket, the female flowers go to seed and shut down. No groping stigmas, no swelling buds, no spicy scent of resin, no rich payload of cannabinoids. No sin semilla, in other words, nothing remotely like it, in any phase of hemp cultivation. Cultivation, then, is the defining difference between marijuana and hemp, but it isn't the only difference.

There are also environmental components. It takes plenty of heat and sunshine, with a particular timing, to produce good marijuana. Until the invention of grow lights, it was almost impossible to grow marijuana in a high-latitude climate like that of Europe. Hemp, yes, all you want. Marijuana, no. That's because the cannabis plant only starts to bloom when the hours of light and darkness equalize at the autumnal equinox. A cannabis plant takes five or six weeks to flower fully, and the more hot, sunny days there are during the plant's flowering, the denser and more resinous the buds become and the more cannabinoids they contain. In fact, the resin may be, among other things, a protection against dehydration, a sort of sunscreen for the plant's delicate reproductive organs. That means that a seed planted in India, for example, or anywhere in the tropics, has a much better chance of developing drug potency compared with an *identical seed* planted in a cool, high-latitude climate where it will grow exuberantly on the long summer days but will blossom only minimally when heat and sun dwindle away quickly after the equinox. That is why we associate marijuana with hot climates in the global south, while the world's chief hemp growing areas, in contrast, are cooler and more northerly.

Finally, although marijuana and hemp have a common origin, there is a genetic difference between them. Contrasting cultivation has created contrasting strains, mutually exclusive populations, as hemp farmers and marijuana farmers worked in isolation from one another over thousands of years. Always, the former selected for tall, strong stems and the latter, for large, resinous buds. The result was a series of strains with genetic endowments distinct enough that they have sometimes been considered separate species. Still, bring them back into geographical proximity with one another, and they cross-pollinate automatically—so much so that, in geographical proximity, they ruin each other by cross-pollinating. For that reason marijuana and hemp do not go together, historically. Europeans and Chinese have grown hemp for many centuries without producing any cannabis drugs, without even realizing, most of the time, that cannabis *could be* a drug.

We have historical snapshots of very separate strains from two famous eighteenth-century botanists. Linnaeus himself described a northern European domestic hemp strain and called it *Cannabis sativa* as part of his new binomial system of scientific nomenclature in the 1750s. A few decades later, another European naturalist, Lamarck, described an Indian drug-producing bush with an almost identical leaf, and believing that it was different enough to constitute a separate species, he named it *Cannabis indica*. (A twentieth-century Russian botanist later described and named an uncultivated ancestral Central Asian variety, *Cannabis ruderalis*.)

There's disagreement, these days, over whether to think of these as distinct species or varieties of a single species, *Cannabis sativa*. Cannabis plants certainly behave as though they are all one species. Why conceptualize as members of different species plants that, under normal conditions, form part of a single sexually

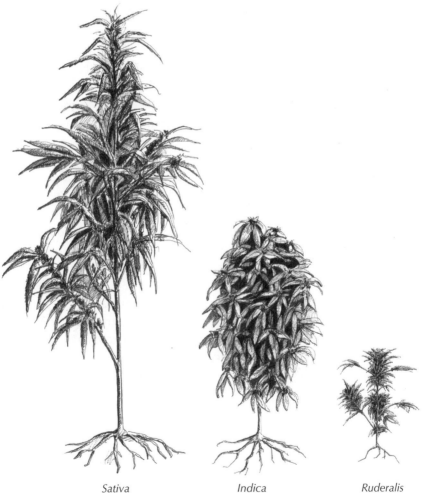

Sativa   Indica   Ruderalis

reproducing population? Any cannabis plant will pollinate any other. Therefore the distinctness of the world's varieties of cannabis has always been provisional, defined by cultivation, maintained by geographical separation, more historical than inherent. Whatever clear distinctions had existed in the 1700s were blurring by the 1800s, as Chinese varieties of hemp were introduced in the United States and Europe. Today distinctions are blurring further as clandestine growers in the United States and Canada, especially, have crossed *sativa* and *indica* strains to make a profusion of hybrids.

The marijuana that first came to the United States around 1900 may have been a hybrid, too. Its origins are somewhat mysterious. Indeed, it seemed to come out of nowhere. The people who brought it from Mexico called it *marihuana*, with an "h," which was the spelling used in the United States until the 1960s and which remains the Spanish-language form of the word. Ironically, the English-language spelling *marijuana*, with a "j," seems to have been established in the 1960s and afterward by people who, like me, thought the "j" looked more authentically Spanish than the "h." Also, a lot of us had heard the story that the word *marijuana* derives from a woman's name, María Juana, which wasn't true but also seemed to favor the "j" spelling. And as long as we're on trivia, sometimes Mexicans called the stuff *grifo*, which is the probable the origin of the "reefer" in *Reefer Madness*.

But let's not get ahead of ourselves. Marijuana became "the world's most used illegal drug" not because of its Mexican origins but because of what happened to it in the United States. So we'll begin our retrospective journey in the twentieth-century United States, before tracing marijuana use back, in successive chapters, to its ultimate origins in prehistoric Central Asia.

2

✳

American Century

Marijuana first appeared in the United States around 1900, a nice round benchmark year. It was a United States newly emerging as a world power because of its victorious 1898 war against Spain, a United States in temporary possession of Cuba and the Philippines, which it had taken from Spain in the war. Internally, this was the eve of the Progressive Era, when confidence in enlightened government action ran high. A "drug-free society," though not a turn-of-the-century term, was one of the era's important goals. The decades-long struggle to eliminate the scourge of alcohol had already triumphed in many state legislatures and was gaining momentum nationally.

Progressives feared the effects of rapid immigration, urbanization, and industrialization that had transformed the United States since the end of its Civil War in 1865. It was a time of labor unrest, and many progressives, who were overwhelmingly white, educated, middle-class, and native-born, felt threatened by the burgeoning population of working-class immigrants and by the formerly enslaved population of southern blacks, some of whom were beginning to move north. They wanted to control the drug use of both groups. The timing of marijuana's arrival in this country with the first appearance of its use by poor black and Mexican migrants was therefore inauspicious, to put it mildly. In progressive eyes, marijuana was a poison, plain and simple.

Many envisioned a titanic global contest among nations, which people of 1900 tended to formulate as a clash of "races." Most progressives thought of the United States as a racially "Anglo-Saxon" nation, currently taking up the "white man's burden" of benevolent world domination ("spreading the benefits of civilization") from a declining Great Britain. Sea power was then the defining military element in geopolitics, and the U.S. military thinking called for U.S. coaling stations in Latin America and Asia, an expanded U.S. Navy, and a Panama Canal to allow quick passage between the Atlantic and Pacific oceans. Coastal defense was no longer the navy's only mission, however. In 1907, Theodore Roosevelt, perhaps the most famous progressive of all, sent a "Great White Fleet" of high seas battleships on a year-long trip around the world "to show the flag."

All this was closely linked to the idea of U.S. trade expansion into Latin America and Asia. Following the severe depression of the 1890s, the captains of U.S. industry agreed that the United States needed to open new export markets to absorb a glut of industrial production that had surged fivefold between 1870 and 1900. Our expanded "blue water" navy was to protect our roving merchant marine fleet as it carried U.S. manufactures around the world. Our acquisition of a naval base on the island of Cuba (Guantánamo Bay) and of Manila's coveted deep-water harbor at the doorstep of China (ah, the fabled Chinese market!) must be understood in this context. And so must the arrival of marijuana as yet another debilitating "vice," a "narcotic" from beyond our shores, eating away at the country's moral fiber . . .

Progressive crusading mentalities shared, as a central tenet, the belief that government action could improve society. Many progressives defined "better" through reference to their Protestant faith. "We stand at Armageddon and we battle for the Lord," intoned Theodore Roosevelt when he became the Progressive Party candidate for president in 1912, and his followers marched around the convention hall singing "Onward Christian Soldiers." Reformers spoke of a "Social Gospel" and of achieving the "Kingdom of

God on Earth." Poisonous drugs had no place in this vision of a society perfectible through idealistic legislation and zealous enforcement. As leading arbiters of moral conscience in the Temperance movement, women had a leading role to play in purifying U.S. society of the most ancient and destructive poison of them all, alcohol. Our great 1919–1933 experiment, Prohibition, was, among other things, quite progressive.

Marijuana was a *minor* poison, by comparison with alcohol, in the eyes of progressive proponents of a drug-free society. The second most important drug historically and in the concern of U.S. progressives was opium, smoked around 1900 by Chinese immigrants and injected by millions of whites as morphine and heroin. Opium was followed, on the alarm scale, by a lesser and much more recent pharmaceutical menace, cocaine, present (like opiates) in many patent medicines, and often associated in the U.S. press with young black men. The most pervasive poisons were those in adulterated foods and medicines, impurities denounced by "muckraking" national magazine journalists. The 1906 Pure Food and Drug Act is a landmark expression of official concern for this toxic environment. The 1914 Harrison Act, the basis for U.S. drug law for many decades, made opiates and cocaine controlled substances, available only by medical prescription. The Eighteenth Amendment and the Volstead Act finished the job, so to speak, by getting alcohol off the streets nationally.

U.S. progressives also projected their reformist impulse internationally, with big implications for the global history of marijuana. People in the U.S.-occupied Philippine Islands consumed large quantities of opium, and because these people were ostensibly being improved and groomed for self-government (the official explanation for our occupation), U.S. authorities extended their anti-poison crusade to colonial Asia, in which they gained the enthusiastic support of Christian missionaries. The U.S. crusade stood in marked contrast to the British example of allowing (when not actively promoting) the Asian opium trade. Zealous U.S. diplomats persevered in a series of international conferences, beginning in the 1909 Shanghai Conference specifically on opium, continuing through the 1920s, and culminating eventually in the UN Single

Convention on Narcotic Drugs of 1961, which extended the current regime of drug control around the world.

Where was marijuana in all of this? The twentieth-century U.S. prohibition of marijuana sprang from an idealist impulse, as well as from religious feeling and a tad of bigotry—but good intentions went awry. Observe.

THE EARLY YEARS

Limited but clear evidence shows that people in the United States first began to smoke marijuana cigarettes on the eve of World War I. These pioneers were laborers recruited in Mexico during the early 1900s to mine ore, maintain railroad tracks, and harvest crops in the western United States. Other migrants soon followed on their own initiative, seeking work. When Mexico's great revolution of 1910 began, the northern part of the country was a major battlefield, dominated by the revolutionary general Pancho Villa. "La Cucaracha," the song famously sung by Villa's followers, refers to marijuana in its lyrics. Ten years of fighting probably encouraged use of marijuana in a militarized Mexico, where it was regarded as a soldier's vice. Meanwhile, noncombatants fled across the border to escape the fighting, often staying with relatives in the United States until it was safe to return home.

The first piece of major historical evidence concerning use of the new drug on this side of the border is an investigation conducted for the U.S. Department of Agriculture in 1917. The investigator reported that marijuana was common in south and west Texas, whether homegrown, brought from Mexico by several companies, or purchased in one-ounce packages from pharmacies and grocery stores, some of which even advertised and sold by mail order. As migrating workers moved north and west from Texas toward the cotton fields and citrus groves of California, into the mining camps of the Rocky Mountain states, and, eventually, into the industrializing cities of the upper Midwest, they took marijuana with them.

It is hard to know what marijuana signified in their lives. Unquestionably, though, its low cost constituted a powerful attraction. Marijuana is naturally an inexpensive crop to grow, store, and transport. A migrant laborer might spend in an afternoon drinking beer money enough to buy marijuana for a month. Only illegality would make marijuana expensive, and it was not yet illegal in the United States. U.S. society as a whole had never heard of marijuana in the 1910s, but Mexican (and Mexican American) society frowned on the drug. They more than frowned. They even endorsed the "reefer madness" image, whereby a few puffs of marijuana could turn anyone at all into a homicidal maniac. The men who actually smoked it obviously knew better, yet social disapproval led them to keep their marijuana out of sight. I say "men" because there are few reports of women smoking it, with the regular exception of prostitutes. We have no good account of marijuana from this first generation of smokers themselves. Middle-class Mexicans and Mexican Americans called them *marihuanos*, a strongly uncompli-mentary term. The state's English-speaking power structure took notice of marijuana only when a fight brought in the police. Such a fight in El Paso, Texas, evidently led, in 1914, to the first municipal ban on marijuana smoking in the United States.

The immigrants often lived isolated in mining camps, railroad boxcars, or the rude housing provided for agricultural migrant laborers. Mainstream white society regarded them with virulent racism. Even when, in the 1920s, they began to find work in cities like Chicago, differences of language, class, and culture limited the social contacts of Mexican migrants. No wonder few whites learned to smoke marijuana from them. Yet someone clearly did learn. The basic U.S. marijuana-smoking customs of the 1960s, such as passing around one cigarette, moistening it with saliva before lighting it, and saving the unsmoked butt to recycle its contents, were unquestionably introduced from Mexico.

Among non-Spanish speakers, those most likely to find them-selves working alongside Mexican immigrants in the 1910s and 1920s were black laborers likewise attracted by marijuana's low cost. Marijuana appeared by 1920 among the black working class in New Orleans, a city in close merchant shipping contact with Mexico. During the first half of the twentieth century, Mexican marijuana represented the great bulk of what was consumed in the

United States, and the consumers were brown or black, generally young and male, too.

Among the blacks were a few hundred musicians who transformed U.S. popular culture in the 1920s, and it is no exaggeration to say that marijuana was part of the process. Jazz music, as it was eventually called, had been created by black musicians in New Orleans at the turn of the century. Before the 1920s, the only way to hear jazz was to go to the poor black dance halls of New Orleans or, famously, its red light districts. Some jazz playing could be heard on Mississippi riverboats that operated upriver, as well. Then came the great migration of southern blacks to the industrial cities of the Midwest and Northeast. New Orleans jazz could then be heard on the South Side of Chicago. Adventurous white working-class young people began to pay attention. New Orleans jazzmen who had moved north to Chicago in the 1920s moved east to New York City in the 1930s. Radio broadcast stations springing up across the country and phonograph discs with one song on each side took jazz to the masses. Jazz was becoming the national sound track, and beyond that, an international sensation of global modernity.

Early jazz music, condemned as lascivious, even infernal, by the older generation, had clear affiliations with youth rebellion. Early jazz was dance music, above all, and U.S. young people succumbed to a notable dance craze in the 1920s. "Modern girls" of the 1920s, dance-floor "flappers," wore their hair short and their skirts high. They might even smoke tobacco and drink illegal liquor, which wasn't hard to find. Alcohol, not marijuana, was the principal intoxicant of the "Jazz Age," perhaps ironically, given that the music's unstoppable rise in popularity coincided with national Prohibition, from 1919 to 1933. Smoking tobacco taught this generation to inhale. Many of the musicians themselves preferred to inhale marijuana, which they most commonly called *reefer*, for reasons that you now understand. Jazz players smoked in and around their performance venues, and often during their practice sessions. A few songs even mention reefer in the title. Whether or not reefer made them play better—they thought so—it made them enjoy playing more. For jazz players, to smoke reefer was to belong to a kind of secret brotherhood. Sometimes they used their elaborate slang, called "jive," to mention reefer (as "muggles," "tea," etc.) onstage, or even on recordings, an inside joke for other "vipers," as they called themselves. Being a viper was part of the jazz players' mystique.

Jazz involved a sort of improvisation and rhythmic "swing" that could not be written down. And never, in the 1920s, could white and black musicians play in the same band, which would have been a sickening outrage according to the dominant racist sensibilities of the day. At first, the only way for whites to learn jazz was to seek out black jazz players, watch them perform night after night, make friends with them, and get some pointers. Eventually, most whites who learned to play jazz did so by wearing out the records of the New Orleans musicians who had created the style, lifting the phonograph needle over and over to repeat a particular passage. Whether in direct association with black jazzmen or by a more remote method, white musicians learned jazz by imitating black musicians. For some, that imitation included reefer.

The association between jazz and marijuana can be exemplified by the most influential trumpet player in global history, Louis Armstrong. Armstrong grew up in the roughest parts of New Orleans and started playing his horn in an institution that was a cross between an orphanage and a reform school. (He was sent there for firing a pistol into the air on the street, a typical expression of high spirits in his neighborhood.) Within a few years, he was part of the first wave of New Orleans musicians to make the move north to Chicago, and in the 1920s his recordings became widely copied models that defined the new musical genre. Armstrong was a lifelong viper who liked his band to practice "high" and who, later in life, after the national ban on marijuana, wrote a letter of protest to President Dwight Eisenhower. By that time, the Federal Bureau of Narcotics kept a file on Armstrong and on many other jazz players.

THE MARIHUANA TAX ACT, 1937

Marijuana was only one of several psychoactive substances legally restricted in the early-twentieth-century United States, as we have seen. When the derivatives of opium poppies and coca leaves became controlled substances in 1915, however, marijuana did not. Unlike cocaine and, especially opiates, the presence of this new poison was incipient, limited, and localized—not yet a national concern. The most abused substance of the early-twentieth-century United States, meanwhile, was unquestionably booze.

Whiskey and hard cider had been omnipresent on the nineteenth-century frontier. Opposition to alcohol use had ebbed and flowed during that century, and many states had banned the sale of the drug well before national Prohibition. Historians agree that, in addition to concerns about the dangers of alcoholism, fears of immigrant drinking figured importantly in the national mood. These were the same years, after all, in which immigration was first restricted by congressional action.

Before national prohibition, a lot of drinking happened in the sort of uproarious saloon familiar to modern viewers from cinematic Westerns. In the industrial north of the United States and in the Midwest, hard-drinking European immigrants frequented saloons, which were also centers for political indoctrination and organizing. This was a period in which European immigrants were suspected of radical doctrines, such as Socialism and Anarchism. More often, the political life of saloons turned on the exchange of votes for benefits, namely, patronage, what these days we call "pork-barrel politics." Saloons seemed a big problem to progressive reformers of the early 1900s. Moreover, whether in Dodge City, Chicago, or Brooklyn, saloons were a man's world, venues in which the only women were prostitutes. The famous activist Carrie Nation believed that she obeyed a higher moral order when she smashed up saloons with an ax. The Women's Christian Temperance Union was an organization of primary importance in building a national consensus for the prohibition of alcohol. In general, the institution of Prohibition in 1919 coincided with, and partly resulted from, a rise in women's political engagement, including a woman's right to vote, and protection of children ranked high among women's goals.

However, the Eighteenth Amendment, outlawing the manufacture, transport, and sale of alcoholic beverages, is the only constitutional amendment ever to be repealed. National prohibition of alcohol soon began to lose popularity because of its mortifying side effects. The saloons disappeared, and consumption of the drug declined by half, but millions of Americans continued to drink. Only the commercialization of alcohol, not its consumption, had been criminalized. The illegal manufacture, transport, and sale of alcohol became a multimillion-dollar business that energized criminals and created a wave of gang violence. The rise of the modern mafia confounded reformers who had promised that controlling drugs would reduce crime. Drinking clubs called "speakeasies" multiplied in place of saloons. Unlike saloons, speakeasies were full of jazz and women who weren't prostitutes, full of gangsters, too, who became jazz connoisseurs and hired many musicians for their late-night carousing. Typically, when the police raided a speakeasy for selling alcohol, they did not arrest the clientele for drinking, which was not illegal per se. Still, people agreed that Prohibition had brought widespread disregard for the law. The moral arguments against alcohol had not changed, but gradually, during the 1930s, our sense of priorities and possibilities had. As the country scraped into the depths of the Great Depression in 1933, it abandoned its "noble experiment" in moral improvement.

Compared to all this, marijuana was hardly an issue in 1933. Most people in the United States did not know what it was. True, its use seems to have risen during the prohibition of alcohol, but mostly among poor black and brown people whose concerns rated little national attention. Still, local lawmakers noticed and reacted. By 1930, marijuana had been prohibited by law in many states, beginning in Texas, California, and other western areas with significant populations of Mexican descent. The creation of state and local laws in the 1920s had elicited very little debate, perhaps none at all. Such laws were advanced as simple matters of public order: "Loco weed," known to drive Mexicans violently and permanently crazy after three puffs, had been outlawed as a public safety measure, end of story. The United States as a whole read the word *marihuana* for the first time in exaggerated newspaper reports that were, in some ways, exceedingly reminiscent of the earlier "temperance noir" stories about violent crimes committed under the influence of "demon rum." Another area of early alarm and

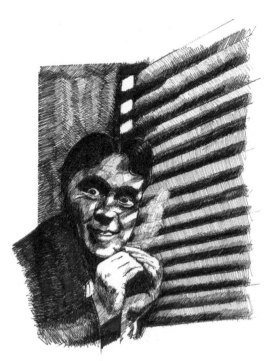

Reefer Madness, *1936.*

prohibition was Louisiana, where the New Orleans commissioner of public safety began a campaign that garnered some national attention. The trouble seems to have started there when a young musician tried to forge a doctor's signature on a prescription for marijuana, which was available in the city for medical use.

More or less at that point, a veteran Prohibition-enforcement agent named Harry Anslinger was appointed head of the newly created National Bureau of Narcotics (FBN). Anslinger was as committed a moral reformer as one could desire. He believed that use of marijuana was wrong and very dangerous. He disliked the black and brown people who used it, and he believed that they were dangerous, too. From the time he became the country's leading narcotics law enforcement officer in 1930, Anslinger worked to raise public awareness of the marijuana menace through systematic publicity. The powerful Hearst newspaper chain, with its strong anti-Mexican attitude, was his staunch ally. Anslinger's anti-marijuana publicity incorporated various sorts of legendary lore and press accounts of sensational crimes, especially those which could be read as threatening "white womanhood." One earnest FBN pamphlet chronicled the marijuana-fueled depredations of a "ginger-colored nigger." Anslinger hated jazz and considered jazz musicians to be corrupters of youth and vectors of the marijuana contagion. He did not single-handedly bring about federal legislation against marijuana, which had already been outlawed in many states, but when the Treasury Department introduced the Marihuana Tax Act in Congress in 1937, Anslinger went to Capitol Hill and made the argument for it.

Anslinger had no real expertise in the matter, and he based his argument on his law-enforcement experience and a few newspaper clippings about ax murders. He was able to pass as an authority on marijuana only because so few people knew or cared about it. Anslinger's authoritative judgment was neither widely informed nor guided by any sort of scientific information. In outlining the marijuana menace, he made no reference to the U.S. government's most careful study of marijuana up to that point, undertaken in 1925 by U.S. Army investigators in the Panama Canal Zone. It is not clear that he had even read the report's conclusion, which found marijuana use to be relatively harmless and had advised *against* prohibiting U.S. soldiers from smoking it. The legislators who passed the Marihuana Tax Act did not require much proof, however, when Anslinger solemnly outlined the threat of "reefer madness." They did not hesitate even when a representative of the American Medical Association impugned the scientific validity of Anslinger's testimony. Even after they voted, some seemed still not quite sure what the insidious and highly addictive new "narcotic" was. But why take a chance, after all, with a drug strongly associated with criminality, blacks, and Mexicans?

The Marihuana Tax Act boldly addressed the problem by making all forms of cannabis effectively illegal nationwide. I say "effectively." Technically the law applied the constitutional power to tax interstate commerce by placing a prohibitively high tax on all sales of cannabis. The law made no distinction between marijuana and hemp. The distinction was not very well understood at the time by anyone involved in lawmaking—and besides, hemp was no longer a major U.S. crop in the 1930s. True, a new processing machine had demonstrated the potential to reinvigorate the crop by making hemp a source of cheap newsprint for the country's myriad daily newspapers. The promise of the new technology prompted an article on the marvels of hemp in a national magazine, *Popular Mechanics*. But agricultural interests did not mount a defense of hemp and, many industries, such as those producing pulpwood and synthetic fibers, had no wish to see hemp reinvigorated. The country as a whole took little notice of the 1937 act, before, during, or for many years after its passage. Even Anslinger experienced an anticlimax. Once he stopped sounding the alarm so vigorously, there proved to be no actual crisis to confront, so he directed his attention to high-profile users, such as Hollywood actors and jazz musicians.

Less than five years after the end of our national crusade against alcohol, the country had taken a momentous step in the direction of future drug wars. But the looming threat, a toxin reputedly inciting murderous "reefer madness," would prove totally bogus.

RISE AND FALL OF THE COUNTERCULTURE

The most notable reaction to the Marihuana Tax Act occurred shortly thereafter in New York City, where mayor Fiorello LaGuardia (who *had* read the Canal Zone report) commissioned a five-year medical, sociological, and criminological study, the first in-depth assessment of marijuana ever done in the United States. Marijuana had been available in New York for about ten years, but the LaGuardia Report found no evidence to support Anslinger's assertion that the new drug was addictive or that it drove users criminally insane. Nor did the study's careful school-by-school survey turn up any indication that marijuana use by schoolchildren constituted a significant problem, despite an alarmist outcry from concerned parents. The researchers were shocked, on the other hand, at how many schoolchildren were starting to smoke tobacco.

They also reported that Harlem and Spanish Harlem were the parts of New York City most affected by marijuana, and that it was associated with jazz venues. A squad of undercover detectives donned pullover sweaters and old shoes to explore the apartments, called "tea pads," where marijuana was smoked socially. Tea pads were characterized by incense, dim lights, furniture to lounge on, and a radio, phonograph, or nickelodeon for music. The detectives found it easy to strike up conversations in a tea pad, where new acquaintances frequently shared cigarettes. Tea-pad denizens liked to philosophize in a manner that the detectives found out of keeping with "the intellectual level" of such persons. Rowdiness was not permitted, nor was sexual activity in evidence, despite the fact that a tea pad's walls were commonly decorated with erotic art, apparently from the *Kama Sutra*. The detectives reported that most people they saw smoking marijuana appeared to be unemployed (this was 1939). Although they did not generalize about smokers' sex or age, arrest figures reveal a clear profile: 90 percent male, 70 percent in their twenties or younger. No surprises there—but interestingly, just under a quarter of those arrested for marijuana were white.

The whites who frequented the tea pads of Harlem in racially segregated New York were the beginnings of a transition. Jazz was still part of what brought adventurous whites across the color line, but now it was also marijuana itself. Here was the contagion that so worried Anslinger. The New York detectives' accounts of tea-induced camaraderie and philosophizing, amid music, incense, and erotic art prefigure the atmosphere of the counterculture. By the late 1940s, a group of writers emerged to give the ethos of the tea pads national projection. Many of these young men had met not far from Harlem, at Columbia University, and all of them were white, as most of their readers and imitators would also be. They prided themselves on their unconventional lifestyles, and that included "tea." Eventually they became known as the Beat-generation writers.

The Beats' interest in jazz and Harlem tea fit easily into their larger rebellion against conventional social norms. They had a taste for Eastern philosophy, sexual experimentation, and mind-altering substances. They somewhat resembled the English Romantic poets—such as Coleridge, Keats, Shelley, and Lord

Byron—whose defiant bohemianism they admired. The most famous Beat writers were the poet Allen Ginsberg (*Howl*, 1956) and
the novelist Jack Kerouac (*On the Road*, 1957). They were nationally influential, but more important than the writers themselves
were the larger phenomena to which they gave voice. The writers were hardly the only young, middle-class whites who had
become sympathetic to black culture, dismissive of mainstream
social norms, and eager to flout them. "Beatniks," the young
admirers of Beat writers, cultivated a distinctive look, including beards, dark sweaters, and sandals—a European appearance
emblematic of their disaffection with U.S. models. Beatniks "got
hip," adopting elements of black slang heard at tea pads. Beatniks
were apt to smoke marijuana, too, perhaps while listening to jazz
or at a poetry reading. At the end of the 1950s, beatniks existed
mostly in a few large cities, notably New York and San Francisco.

Like the Beat writers, these new marijuana-smoking cultural
dissidents were apt to be white and middle-class. Their marijuana
smoking became independent of tea pads run by, and mostly for,
African Americans. But the rarity of beatniks—most people in the
United States never laid eyes on one except in a magazine—made
them remote and not very menacing. Then the Sixties happened.
By the 1970s, the lonely cultural dissidence represented by 1950s
beatniks had become a mass phenomenon and defined the intervening decade—all, it seemed to some, in a cloud of marijuana
smoke.

To understand the rise of marijuana smoking as a mass phenomenon in the 1960s, one must begin by observing the wave
that buoyed it up. The great demographic wave created by the
post–World War II baby boom swept into high school and college in the early 1960s. Youth itself, not childhood, but embattled
adolescence and headstrong young adulthood, set the tone for the
decade. Youth rebellion is a recurring phenomenon in history, but
far from a universal one. Most of the time, young people seem
willing to obey the norms and the leadership established by their
elders. Rapid social change tends to undermine the authority of
age and wisdom, however. The 1920s had displayed elements of
youth rebellion, as we have seen. The 1930s, though not a decade

of generational rebellion, had contributed to the development of a distinct youth culture because, in the absence of employment opportunities, young people spent more years in school associating primarily with their peers. Then, what the Depression did for high school attendance, post–World War II economic recovery and prosperity did for college attendance. More peer culture. Postwar prosperity helped young people to develop their separate cultural identity—the sense that they did not share their parents' values and tastes—through more intensive consumption of age-specific clothing and entertainment. This greater feeling of separateness, when combined with youthful assertiveness and resources, made challenges to age and authority notably common in the 1950s. "What are you rebelling against?" someone asks Marlon Brando in a 1953 movie. "Whattaya got?" he replies. A notable 1955 youth movie was *Rebel without a Cause*. Causes aplenty soon appeared.

Civil rights, for one. The dramatic early struggles for African American civil rights occurred just at this time. After fighting against Nazi racism, the United States as a nation had begun to look at southern segregation more critically. In 1954, the U.S. Supreme Court disallowed the "separate but equal" rationalization of segregation, and soon the Montgomery bus boycott was under way. Martin Luther King Jr. emerged to lead a national movement that had a moral superiority obvious to everyone except southern whites personally invested in segregation. The movement gained national momentum, presidential support, world attention. In the early 1960s, university students from the north participated in "Freedom Rides" and voter registration campaigns in southern states. Those inspired by this cause learned to apply the tactic of civil disobedience, calmly resisting sheriff's deputies in Mississippi or Alabama in the name of a higher moral authority. Most of these students had probably never tried marijuana, but the experience certainly suggested to them that not all laws merited obedience.

Soon many would decide that, by the same token, not all wars merited patriotic support. Vietnam divided the country infinitely more than later conflicts in Iraq and Afghanistan. A New Left of student radicals appeared, focused not so much, like the "Old" Left, on organized labor, but rather, on questioning the anti-Communist consensus of U.S. Cold Warriors. The beyond-liberal Students for a Democratic Society, the national face of the New Left, was founded in 1962. During that same year, the Cuban Missile Crisis reminded the country of the threat of nuclear annihilation—a product of "old-style" thinking, said the young radicals. In 1965, the United States began the rapid escalation of its military involvement in Vietnam that led to the deployment of troops. In 1966, students acquired a more immediate reason to question the war when the government stopped issuing automatic draft deferments to university students. To students who opposed the war for whatever reason, the idea of being drafted and sent to fight against their will provoked angry protest. In the late 1960s, student protesters occupied buildings on university campuses and organized major demonstrations around the country.

A *counter*culture was emerging. As with the civil rights movement, resistance to the Vietnam War encouraged a spirit of moral outrage among its participants, a feeling of alienation and opposition toward not just a particular policy but an entire social, political, and cultural system, which protesters called "The Establishment," "The System," or even, for lack of anything more specific, "The Status Quo." There were no more rebels without a cause. Various sorts of dissidence coalesced in a general attitude of opposition and protest. Opposition to the war in Vietnam went together with youth, a general proclivity to question social norms, support for civil rights, and a respect for expressions of black culture, which was part of a general interest in the world's poor and downtrodden. The counterculture was not served à la carte. Rather, it was a package deal, a group identity, a tribe.

The clearest personifications of that tribe were called "hippies" in a San Francisco newspaper, and the name stuck. It referred to the hip slang spoken by San Francisco beatniks who were colonizing a run-down neighborhood called Haight-Ashbury. "If you're going to San Francisco," counseled the pop anthem of 1967, "be sure to wear some flowers in your hair." Many thousands of young people went to Haight-Ashbury from across the United States to become hippies without knowing much more than that song. It wouldn't be hard to find hippies, because you knew them when you saw them. Long hair made boys into hippies, as did faded blue jeans, and the general look of a homeless waif. And sometimes no underwear. "Hippie chicks" wore long "granny" dresses from the used clothing store, without makeup or bras or, possibly, shoes. Both sexes wore Native American beadwork, South American fabrics, and African motifs. Most controversially, some hippies wore clothing made out of the national flag or fabric resembling it. That produced an angry reaction, as did a number of other hippie traits. Hippies advocated "Peace and Love," and pacifism seemed unpatriotic and effeminate to many Americans during the Vietnam War. Hippie love was *brotherly* love, of course, directed to those on whom one refused to make war, but it was also *free* love. Make love, not war! Middle America, as it was then called, looked on hippie promiscuity with horror. Hippies seldom bathed, commented "straight" America. And they wanted to live like "bums," without working! Many other hippie traits were controversial, too. Hippies scorned material things—theoretically, at any rate—and they might live without furniture, sleeping on mattresses on the floor. They prized living spontaneously, making do creatively without a silly full-time job, drifting here and there, hitchhiking or traveling in an old Volkswagen bus, a life "on the road." This fantasy of carefree poverty was contradicted, of course, and also facilitated, by the social origins of these young people. Hippies were only poor, for the most part, when in conflict with their suburban parents.

Finally, there were drugs, of course. Hippies frowned on alcohol, which they associated with loutish violence and lack of imagination, but they were open to anything else. Marijuana was by far the most popular choice, but there were also pharmaceutical "uppers" and "downers" that had been widely consumed for years, and several sorts of hallucinogenic drugs: psilocybin (from "magic" mushrooms), mescaline (from peyote cactus), and laboratory-synthesized LSD, lysergic acid diethylamide, "acid" for short. The point was to try them and see what one preferred. But the hallucinogens—of which marijuana was the mildest and LSD the most powerful—held a special countercultural significance because of their reputed mind-expanding qualities. They were believed to "deprogram" people made "robotic" by pervasive mass media of

"The System," allowing them to experience the world in a manner unfiltered by cultural conditioning. For crusaders who believed that mind-altering drugs were the key to a better world, deprogrammed *ex*-robots would recover their human potential. They would be able to see through the myriad forms of social manipulation, resist the bombardment of media messages to conform and consume. True believers thought that the truth would simply be unveiled to the mind of the LSD users. They would automatically perceive the senselessness of War, the sacredness of Nature, the brotherhood of Man. Half a century later, one notices immediately that a deprogrammed robot will require *re*-programming if it is to function at all. The CIA took the idea of deprogramming seriously as a potential weapon in the Cold War, conducting experiments with LSD and other drugs.

It wasn't alone in its interest. From 1961 to 1963, Harvard psychology professor Timothy Leary conducted deprogramming experiments with prison inmates before leaving the university to promote the life-changing insights that, according to him and his Harvard associate Richard Alpert, could be gained from LSD. Oregon novelist Ken Kesey first tried LSD as a volunteer subject in a CIA study, then began to promote LSD use on the fringes of the Stanford University community. Neither Leary nor Kesey had university support, but both men developed personal followings and—Leary especially—considerable news coverage. A single droplet of LSD will send those who ingest it on a six-to-eight-hour "trip" that can be very frightening. Kesey's "Merry Pranksters" wore costumes, drove around in a party-colored bus, and liked to dose the unsuspecting with "electric Kool-Aid." Of the various drugs favored by the counterculture, LSD was the most likely to produce a philosophical epiphany of some kind, but LSD trips could traumatize the tripper, and daily use of it was infrequent. If hallucinogens were the hard liquor of hippie life, reserved for special occasions, then marijuana was more like hippie beer, an enhancing accompaniment to daily activities.

Much more than LSD, therefore, marijuana became a touchstone of countercultural belonging, a lot more fun than the hard stuff, yet still a hallucinogen. Crusaders like Leary and Kesey, and also

Allen Ginsberg, certainly believed that marijuana helped build the counterculture. Ginsberg's highly visible 1966 article in the *Atlantic Monthly* argued that the effects of marijuana encouraged users to turn away from discursive thinking (the result of social programming) and toward spontaneous, creative interpretations of direct sensory experience. By that time, the major national upsurge in pot smoking had clearly begun. The steep increase in marijuana use among university students, particularly, occurred following the LSD-oriented "Human Be-In," a 1967 San Francisco gathering of possibly twenty thousand at which Leary and Ginsberg were featured speakers; Kesey, already pursued by the FBI, was present incognito.

Unquestionably, marijuana and LSD often altered the worldview of those who used them. They were, at a minimum, unsettling experiences. Leary's famous formula, "Turn On, Tune In, and Drop Out," the keynote of the "Human Be-In," was a program for personal revolution that started with drugs ("turning on"), proceeded through acquisition of new values and self-knowledge ("tuning in"), and culminated with a principled rejection of existing social practices ("dropping out"), preferably in a communal living arrangement. Not all who turned on really tuned in, and few, indeed, went so far as to drop out.

There is no reason to doubt, though, that daily use of marijuana alienated many people from prevailing social norms. To become a "pothead" made a big difference in one's life. To begin with, possession of marijuana made you, ipso facto, a criminal. Hippies, or anybody else who carried a rolled-up plastic sandwich bag with an ounce or so, ten-dollars' worth, of Mexican marijuana learned to think of themselves as outlaws and of the police as enemies. On the positive side, not a few people noticed that getting high enhanced their sexual activities, especially, for men, by delaying orgasm. A notable hippie taste for the zany and the outrageous does not seem un-drug-related, either. The Youth International Party (YIP), which chose its name mostly so that its members could call themselves Yippies, and which basically thought of itself as the political arm of hippiedom, lightheartedly made fun of itself and the U.S. military when, during one protest, Yippies tried to levitate the Pentagon. In an iconic photograph of the day, a hippie chick places a flower in the rifle barrel of a soldier sent to quell the disturbance. The 1960s vogue for "psychedelic" or surrealist visual art that mimics hallucinations also reflected an interest in altered states of consciousness. The unsettling effect of mind-altering substances prompted some to become spiritual seekers. Countercultural "gurus" studied Buddhism, visited India, and advocated transcendental meditation. Eastern philosophy gained a greater currency than ever before in American life. The psychedelic experience also provoked, in many people, an embrace of mysticism, such as the vogue for astrology. Until the "Age of Aquarius" of the 1960s, the zodiac was for gypsy fortune tellers and their clients.

Music gave countercultural drug use international projection. "Sex, drugs, and rock and roll" went together. As in the Jazz Age, the musicians producing the most popular music of the 1960s referred to drugs in their song lyrics and used marijuana while composing, practicing, and performing. This was true of headliners like Bob Dylan, the Rolling Stones, and the Beatles, and it was true of many small fry, too. For the band called the Grateful Dead, who emerged from the San Francisco hippie scene around 1965 and spent the next three decades touring almost nonstop, drug use was an encouraged form of audience participation. Rock concerts were commonly accompanied by psychedelic light shows designed to mimic and enhance visual hallucinations. Marijuana smoking became especially de rigueur at the open-air rock festivals that brought together tens, or sometimes hundreds, of thousands of young people. Feeling strength in numbers, attendees smoked marijuana openly and shared it with those around them. The 1969 Woodstock Music and Art Festival in New York State was the largest and most famous of these. Despite rampant drug use among the half million attendees, the organizers proudly pointed out, no one got hurt. The same could not be said, however, about the Altamont Free Concert held near San Francisco later that year, which was billed as Woodstock West. There, the performers' ill-chosen "body guards" (members of the Hell's Angels motorcycle gang) killed an apparently inebriated young man who brandished a pistol and tried to climb onstage during a performance by the Rolling Stones.

Altamont seemed to crystallize a national reaction against the counterculture. Soon, the Sixties were over. All the in-your-face hippie disrespect for traditional values, the brazen burning of draft cards and flags—but not bras, although the legend continues—had stoked the anger of those who identified with those values. The 1968 murders of Martin Luther King Jr. and Robert Kennedy, grim reminders of JFK's traumatic 1963 assassination, had particularly shocked the nation. Neither event was linked to the counterculture, but both fueled a fear that things were spinning out of control. Militant "Black Power" had overshadowed the cause of black civil rights, with its stubbornly nonviolent, hymn-singing marches. The last years of the 1960s were punctuated by race riots and angry, ongoing protests against the Vietnam War, including the disruption of Chicago's 1968 Democratic National Convention by Yippies and other demonstrators. Students seized buildings at major universities and were besieged by the police, making "campus unrest" a grave concern in national polls. Pollution and the overall health of the natural environment had become a concern for the first time, too, thanks partly to countercultural "tree-hugging." In 1969, the nation contemplated the bizarre murders committed by the so-called Manson family, a California hippie commune run by a psychopath who based his apocalyptic prophecies on the lyrics of Beatles songs. In New York City, the colorfully named Stonewall Riots launched what would become Gay Liberation. Some thought they beheld the new Sodom and Gomorrah, others the dawn of the promised revolution. Both were disappointed.

Marijuana's sudden new prominence in the 1960s stemmed from a radically changed view of it. The idea of murderous "reefer madness" had been abandoned by critics and totally inverted by exponents of countercultural "peace and love." But when reaction swept the country, as it soon did, ideas about marijuana changed again.

DRUG WAR, CULTURE WAR

For good or ill, the Age of Aquarius did not much outlast the 1960s. The United States gradually withdrew its soldiers from Vietnam, disorder in the streets abated, LSD use dwindled. Marijuana smoking did not decline much, if any, however. Tens of millions of young Americans had tried marijuana, and many of them continued to smoke it throughout their lives, yet marijuana remained illegal. After Aquarius came the War on Drugs.

The counterculture expanded its numbers but softened its focus in the 1970s as it branched out from cities like San Francisco and New York to the rest of the nation. Images of hippies and demonstrators had repelled many, perhaps most, U.S. viewers, especially in rural, religious, conservative communities, but they had inspired millions of others to imitation. In the 1970s, countercultural attitudes, activities, and attire appeared in every U.S. city, marijuana smoking notably among them.

Marijuana use continued the general pattern established in the 1960s. It was most common in people's late teens and early twenties; in that age range about 40 percent of the population had tried it. Habitual daily users constituted only about a tenth of that number. In addition, marijuana had spread pervasively into walks of life far from hippiedom. State anti-marijuana laws underwent limited liberalization, and the National Organization for the Reform of Marijuana Laws (NORML) campaigned confidently. It seemed only a matter of time until full legalization. Convenience stores around the country stocked new brands of cigarette papers that everyone well knew were exclusively for marijuana. "Head shops," heavy with incense, offered all the imaginable paraphernalia of marijuana smoking except for the substance itself. Meanwhile, national clothing chains advertised their own awkward versions of hippie-influenced fashions. Some remaining hippies, in search of authenticity, shifted from psychedelic to homespun motifs and invented "country rock."

As the decade advanced, the national spotlight turned away from what remained of the counterculture, which began to appear not so apocalyptic after all. The bicentennial celebration of national independence in 1976, with its patriotic sparkle, seemed a sign of the changing times. Any sense of a unified movement to reinvent society evaporated in this process of diffusion and co-optation. Now it *was* counterculture à la carte, which meant, increasingly, no longer a brotherhood, not really a culture, at all. Gradually, even youthful rebellion itself abandoned the counterculture, as former hippies cut their hair, concentrated on careers, and raised children who aspired to attend the high school prom in limousines. Whatever mystique marijuana had once possessed as a mind-expanding drug evaporated, too.

By the 1980s, the counterculture was "history." True enough, countercultural attitudes such as environmentalism and women's equality and, more gradually, liberty of sexual orientation had been embraced by the country as a whole. Mainstream newspapers now published your horoscope. But in overall style and tone, the 1980s seemed the antithesis of the 1960s, as 1980s children reacted against the iconoclasm of their parents' generation. Modish youth, distressingly including one's own children, now admired conservative "success" and desired, without embarrassment, to emulate the rich and famous. The unthinkable, from my perspective, had happened. Conservatism had become *cool*. Wall Street investment bankers and venture capitalists took on hero status in popular culture. Cultural opposition and young rebellions continued, of course, now with purple-haired, nihilistic "punk" stylings, but as an undercurrent only. The urban poor became an *underclass* that lost its claim on our collective conscience. National politics expressed the country's predominantly conservative mood. Southern whites angered by the civil rights movement moved solidly into the Republican Party, which was also buoyed up, in the 1980s and 1990s, by fervent evangelical Christians all over the United States.

Strong anti-drug attitudes predominated in 1980s public discourse, which focused on public health and the social costs of drug abuse. Even alcohol and tobacco became the object of greater restrictions. "Fetal alcohol syndrome" entered our everyday vocabulary, replacing the idea that beer encourages lactation. Drunk driving, a practice as old as driving itself, became the object of highly successful public safety campaigns that taught partiers to "designate" a driver. An awareness of the health risks that smoke creates for nonsmokers dramatically reduced the acceptability of cigars and cigarettes in bars, restaurants, and people's houses. Protection of children was a persuasive argument in many of these cases.

Meanwhile, the War on (illegal) Drugs, first "declared" by Richard Nixon in the early 1970s, intensified. In 1986, Ronald Reagan further institutionalized it by ordering that all executive agencies of the federal government implement drug-testing programs, and the next year, when a train wreck in Maryland was attributed to the engineer's marijuana use, private companies implemented routine drug testing nationwide. Other illicit drugs upstaged marijuana in the public eye, though. First in prominence were the refined alkaloids of the Andean coca plant, cocaine and "crack." Cocaine was 1980s chic, enormously expensive, suitable to the high-rolling ("if you've got it, flaunt it") lifestyle of a young stockbroker. Crack, the cheaper and more potent down-market version of the drug, however, was associated with crime-ridden slums. Illegal manufacture of methamphetamine, "crystal meth" or "crank," gained traction among rural whites. None of these drugs had any countercultural chops. They were about the way they felt, period. The new "youth drug," MDMA, a pharmaceutical amphetamine called Ecstasy, did have a touch of utopian mystique. A powerful euphoriant, Ecstasy gained its glamour from close association with the impromptu all-night dance events called "raves," but it never gained wide currency, despite its appealing name.

How could it? High crime rates were generating colossal alarm, and drugs and crime seemed inseparable to the general public. Several presidents saw fit to appoint a federal "Drug Czar" with nebulous powers. In the 1980s and 1990s, U.S. politicians found that voters habitually rewarded tough talk about the War on Drugs, and they delivered plenty of "tough-on-drugs" legislation. The result was a series of mandatory minimum sentencing guidelines that produced more, and longer, prison terms for convicted drug users and shifted effective sentencing power from judges to prosecutors. The tough-on-drugs sentencing guidelines overloaded U.S. prisons while doing little to reduce the availability of any kind of illegal substance. Marijuana smokers continued to number in the millions, but they had hunkered down. Until the campaign for what became California's Compassionate Use Act of

1996, the only public advocates of legalizing cannabis pretended to be interested primarily in hemp.

Still, millions were smoking marijuana, and demand begets supply. That supply still came mostly from abroad. In the 1990s, the drug wars were fought increasingly outside the United States, in Latin American countries colonized or traversed by a burgeoning illegal drug traffic. Through the 1960s, most of the U.S. marijuana supply crossed the border from Mexico in cars and trucks driven by small-scale amateur smugglers. In the 1970s, the U.S. government policed the border more rigorously and, with the collaboration of the Mexican government, had marijuana crops south of the border sprayed aerially with a defoliant called paraquat. As sales of Mexican marijuana dropped, Jamaican and Colombian entrepreneurs saw a lucrative business opportunity and took over the traffic to an extent that, by 1980, Colombia had become the world's leading exporter of marijuana. Colombian marijuana was notably superior and more costly. Most Colombian marijuana came into the United States across the Caribbean, by air and by sea, until U.S. military interdiction of Caribbean routes forced the traffic back into Mexico (and later Central America). Cocaine, far more valuable by weight, became the preferred commodity of Colombian traffickers. The rise of competing drug mafias (called cartels in the United States) took a grievous toll, but that toll was remote from U.S. consumers. What they did feel was the higher price. The steadily rising price of marijuana inspired more domestic production, a significant portion of it hidden away under grow lights in closets, attics, and basements. By 2000, the formerly disparaged "homegrown" item had been thoroughly gentrified and replaced by pampered *sin semilla* in an array of prized hybrids usually cloned from cuttings, rather than grown from seed, to retain the special attributes of name-brand strains.

In the new millennium, the erstwhile mind-expanding drug of the counterculture had become a pitfall for unmotivated adolescents, a comforting palliative for the gravely ill, even a legal recreational euphoriant for upscale blue-state consumers, and yet, somehow, in other states, it remained a relentlessly outlawed substance that still landed millions in jail. Where was the logic?

NEWS FLASH

Marijuana never was a devil weed that drove people violently insane after three puffs. The 1936 *Reefer Madness* image of the drug seemed hysterically wrong by century's end. But the idea that pot was an inherently mind-expanding drug had also more or less vanished, lingering only as quaint hippie lore. Evidently, it had been the critique of racism, religion, sexuality and gender, consumer capitalism, and patriotic warfare that expanded the minds of 1960s pot smokers and led them to question The Status Quo. Without such tea-pad philosophizing, marijuana had come to seem just another feel-good recreational drug.

Meanwhile, by 2000 the U.S. counterculture and its aftermath had totally altered marijuana's global status. Young American dissidents had introduced the drug to their British counterparts almost from the start, as symbolized by Dylan's "turning on" the Beatles at New York's Delmonico Hotel in 1964. Media coverage of the counterculture, and especially its music, gave marijuana a globally projected glamour that stimulated its use among European, Asian, and Latin American young people affluent enough to emulate U.S. lifestyles. During the 1970s, once U.S. soldiers had enthusiastically embraced the drug in Vietnam, their Cold War deployment around the world played a part, too, in the transnational dissemination of marijuana. In sum, the counterculture had made marijuana "the world's most used illegal drug," something it was far from being in 1900.

As coming chapters move outward from the United States and backward in time, we will discover a very different and little-known global history of marijuana, a history defined, most often, by the social identity of the users. The poor, migrating marijuana users of the early-twentieth-century United States will turn out to be typical of the last few centuries. However, the idea shared by 1920s jazz vipers, 1950s beatniks, and 1960s hippies, who associated the drug with creative, unconventional thinking, has even stronger precedents in global history, as we will see.

If marijuana came to the United States from Mexico, Jamaica, and Colombia, how was it being used *there*? Latin America and the Caribbean—parts of the Atlantic World created by Europeans, Africans, and Native Americans beginning around 1500—constitute the least-understood locales on the drug's historical itinerary.

3

✳

Atlantic World

The 1910s and 1920s "outbreak" of marijuana in the United States was, in effect, an extension of Mexico's outbreak a few decades earlier, and Mexican marijuana, almost exclusively, supplied the U.S. market through the 1960s. Colombia became a major supplier of marijuana to U.S. consumers in the 1970s. By that time, U.S. soldiers and vacationers in Panama, Costa Rica, Brazil, and Jamaica had learned that marijuana was also available in those places. So what is the history of marijuana in Latin America?

There is no overview of the subject in any language. This gap in the global history of marijuana is only beginning to be filled by careful research, and a major mystery still remains. Cannabis is clearly not native to the Americas. No form of it existed in the Western Hemisphere before European colonization created an interconnected "Atlantic World" around 1500. European hemp, the *Cannabis sativa* that the colonizers introduced throughout their American colonies, had never been used to get high. When marijuana smoking started in Mexico and, then, the United States, it seemed totally disconnected from Old World drug traditions—so much so, that it took years for the world to realize that New World marijuana was a form of Old World cannabis. Where did psychoactive marijuana come from?

HEMP AND RUM, STRATEGIC RESOURCES

To start to untangle this mystery, let's take a closer look at hemp, the cannabis that the Europeans brought with them.

Although hemp fiber has numerous applications, one of them—hemp for the sails, rigging, and other cordage needed by sailing ships—towers over others in global history. Beginning when early Mediterranean seafarers established the first maritime trade routes, right down to the rise of steam power and the decline of wind navigation in the late 1800s, hemp was the preferred material for sails and cordage in the global West. Hemp fibers are extremely long, which means that the rope and sails made from them can possess great tensile strength without being excessively heavy. Imagine the need for strength when sea winds filled a billowing sail to drive a hundred-ton vessel through heavy seas. Imagine the advantages of light weight when sailors clambered aloft to reef sails soaked with rain. Flax was second best, and after cotton gins began mechanical processing of cotton in the early 1800s, making it less expensive, cotton too went into sailcloth. Today, "canvas" is a heavy fabric made of cotton, suitable for a ship's sail. But the word *canvas*, virtually a synonym for sail, comes from the word *cannabis*.

Cotton sails were still a thing of the future when, in the 1500s, various European countries—principally Portugal, Spain, France, and England—competed with one another to establish seaborne empires. In fact, it is not an exaggeration to say that European monarchies wanted overseas colonies, in part, so that they could plant hemp there. Large navies and merchant fleets meant building and rigging thousands of ships, and it meant repeating that process every few years as hulls got leaky and sails and rigging wore out. Maritime construction denuded parts of the European countryside, and it made new demands on European fiber crops, flax and hemp. It has been calculated that to fully rig a single large European sailing ship required as much as 90 tons of hemp, produced on 450 acres of land. Early modern European forests dissolved into planks and masts, and competing countries needed a lot more hemp than they had grown traditionally. In England, Elizabeth I mandated that landowners with sixty acres or more all plant hemp. Early

English colonists at Jamestown, Virginia, and New Plymouth, Massachusetts, were asked to plant hemp, too. To encourage production, a number of English colonies in North America allowed partial payment of taxes in hemp fiber. Both the Portuguese and the Spanish eventually established government hemp plantations in their American colonies.

Hemp was not just a strategic resource, either. It was also a routine part of life in the interconnected societies that composed the Atlantic World. Any farmer on either shore of the Atlantic Ocean, after 1500, might well grow some hemp for domestic use. Fine fabrics, called linens, could be made of hemp as well as flax. The "homespun" clothing of the North American frontier was normally spun (and woven and stitched) at home using hemp fiber. Harvesting and processing hemp fiber was labor-intensive and never mechanized. To derive the necessary raw material from the harvested plant, one first let it lie in the field to "rot," for a time, so that the softer tissue would decompose, then stacked it to dry, then thrashed it manually against a wooden frame to extract the billowy fibers of extraordinary length. One could then make a rope or a cinch, or a pair of pants, and if any fiber were left over, apply it to one's taxes or barter it for something else. Because hemp fiber was valuable, not perishable, easy to store and transport, and always in high demand, store owners were often happy to take it in trade. In the Atlantic World, people made rope in a long structure called a "rope walk," where workers paced hundreds of feet back and forth on a covered walkway, twisting hemp fibers. Kentucky, on the remote trans-Appalachian frontier, had hundreds of them.

European hopes of a colonial hemp bonanza were disappointed, however. America never became a major supplier of hemp for Europe's strategic maritime needs. The lands around the Baltic Sea, Russia especially, remained the best source of high-quality blond hemp fiber, produced by methods much more complex than field rotting. New England, with its significant shipping industry, had to import hemp fiber from overseas. In the early 1800s, Kentucky became the one part of the New World to see spontaneous development of commercial hemp production. But field-rotted Kentucky hemp was of such poor quality that even the U.S. Navy preferred to import the more expensive Russian product. Eventually, the main market for Kentucky hemp fiber, once it had been woven into rough cloth, was on slave-driving plantations that employed it to wrap bales of cotton for shipment to market in Europe. The Kentucky workers who sowed, harvested, and processed the hemp crop were themselves slaves, and hemp declined in importance as a U.S. crop after the abolition of slavery, mostly because the age of sail was ending.

In sum, marijuana's homely sibling, hemp, played a crucial supporting role in one of global history's defining events: European seaborne exploration and colonization of America, Africa, and parts of Asia between 1500 and 1900. But that role had nothing whatsoever to do with psychoactive properties. Europeans seem never to have tried to smoke their cannabis crop in this time period. People in Africa definitely did. Therefore, it makes sense to ask whether any slaves in the U.S. South—perhaps in, say, Kentucky—smoked cannabis. If they had been familiar with cannabis at home, after all, why not sample the domestic variety in Virginia or Maryland? For whatever reason, despite claims to the contrary, smoking hemp was never a general practice among blacks, whites, or anybody else in the United States before 1900. On the other hand, the European colonizers of the New World were definitely hard-drinking people, which brings us to a second great strategic resource of the Atlantic World in the 1600s, 1700s, and 1800s: ethanol.

Ethanol is natural alcohol, the product of fermentation, a metabolic process by which yeast breaks down sugar, the fructose in grapes, for example. But ethanol-producing bacteria stop producing ethanol when the concentration gets beyond 12 to 13 percent, limiting the potency of fermented beverages such as beer and wine. To make stronger liquor requires distillation, technologically a more involved process. Distillation was known to the ancient Greeks and, then, during the medieval period, to the Arabs, who preserved ancient learning that was lost in medieval Europe. But distillation was merely a toy of experimental scientists until around 1500, when Germans began to distill wine to make brandy, a word meaning "burnt wine." This new fire water was so much more potent than fermented drinks that contemporaries were not sure they relied on the same active ingredient.

Europe's capitalist economic growth in the centuries after 1500 turned distillation into a drug revolution. For centuries, Europeans had drunk as much beer and wine as they could produce, which seemed never to be enough. As subsistence-oriented medieval Europe became market-oriented early modern Europe, traditional scarcities gave way to capitalist surpluses. Surplus grain was preserved and put to use through fermentation. (Grain must be malted, to make it sweet, before fermenting, though.) Surplus wine was preserved by distilling it. The Germans who started making brandy did so partly because they had surplus wine on hand. The colonization of the Americas brought new forms of abundance to Europeans, most notably, for our story, the creation of sugarcane plantations in Brazil and the Caribbean. The basic raw material for ethanol had always been in rather short supply in Europe. In the 1600s, though, colonial sugar arrived in Europe's Atlantic ports by the crate, along with a distilled liquor made from it, rum. In the 1700s, English landowners found a market for their surplus grain with distillers eager to make gin. Grain-based distillation further fueled trade and the growth of market capitalism and, thus, European seaborne expansion.

One of the peculiarities of European seaborne expansion was the large role of small trading nations. Tiny Portugal pioneered sail navigation of the African coast, initiated the Atlantic slave trade, and established a seaborne merchant empire that stretched from Brazil to the Indian Ocean, China, Japan, and Indonesia. Through the 1500s, Portuguese ships maintained something close to a trading monopoly in Africa and Asia. Then other small, maritime countries of Europe took their turns at strutting on a global stage. The Dutch, particularly, made distillation a strategic asset in their brief bid for world domination. Their drug of choice at home was beer, but beer (being difficult to preserve and transport) was not yet a practical commodity for long-distance trade, and Holland was all about trade. As a historic center of the European wine trade, it was a good place to distill wine into brandy. The canny Dutch therefore realized multiple advantages in commercializing hard liquor.

Simply because they were more concentrated, brandy, rum, gin, and other distilled spirits got customers drunk faster and kept them drunk longer. That gave them five to ten times the value, by weight and bulk, of fermented drinks—a crucial consideration in long-distance trade. Furthermore, liquor could be stored almost indefinitely and it improved with age, likewise facilitating its commercialization. As a result, the amount of alcohol consumed by Europeans rose alarmingly. London, especially, experienced a "gin craze" from 1700 to 1750, involving a scale and intensity of alcoholism and related social pathologies never before witnessed in modern history.

The English, too, made of distilled spirits a strategic trading resource. English colonials distilled rum from abundant Caribbean sugar and whiskey from even-more-abundant American corn. Rum-making in prosperous Boston, Providence, and Philadelphia was part of the "triangular" slave trade, a historical pattern that brings the entire Atlantic World into view more or less as follows. Yankee traders took cloth and guns to trade for slaves on the African coast, carried the slaves to Caribbean islands covered with sugarcane plantations, traded the slaves for sugar, and sailed home to make rum and count their profits. English settlers also traded distilled spirits to Native Americans. The aboriginal natives of the United States and Canada were a global rarity, people whose traditional cultures did not include any significant use of ethanol, which, in its highly concentrated form, hit them more or less like a speeding truck. The Europeans, well aware of the drug's devastating impact on the Indians, sometimes supplied it with that very end in mind.

Hemp and rum, then, played notable parts in creating the Atlantic World of 1500 to1900. Meanwhile, where was marijuana?

MEXICO, AND A MYSTERY

One place it was, we can say with certainty, was Mexico—acquiring the name that migrating workers later introduced to the United States. The origin of the word *marijuana* is clearly Mexican. It may derive from the Mexican tendency to use the name María as a verbal disguise for hallucinogenic substances that were condemned by the Catholic Church. Hallucinogenic peyote, for example, was called Santa Rosa María; another mild hallucinogen, María Santísima. Marijuana wasn't named for a soldier's sweetheart, María Juana, as the story goes. Such overtly specific origin stories are almost never true. But María Juana certainly *was* another verbal disguise for the drug. Moreover, soldiers' sweethearts do figure prominently in the story of marijuana, and so does the disapproval of the Catholic Church. Much remains unknown, however. A dearth of information is, alas, a constant in the global history of cannabis before 1900.

The historical contrast with evidence on alcohol (and tobacco) is quite astounding. Spanish archives groan under the weight of records relating to alcohol and tobacco in the New World. Unlike the Indians of what is now the United States and Canada, the Aztecs (and their related subject peoples) made and drank ethanol. By Aztec law, the common people drank only (and then, heavily) on ritual occasions. Pulque, fermented from the juice of the maguey cactus, was their wine, and the common people of Mexico continued to drink pulque for centuries. The Spanish rulers of colonial Mexico lamented the large consumption of pulque and taxed every ounce of it, very lucratively indeed—the reason for all those archived official records. Something similar could be said about tobacco, its pre-Columbian origins, its ritual significance, its many users in the colonial period, its lucrative tax revenues. Cigarettes (wrapped in paper, as opposed to cigars, wrapped in tobacco leaves) were seemingly invented in Mexico and mass-produced there, for the first time anywhere, in the 1700s.

In comparison, the total of what is known about the history of marijuana in Mexico before 1850 would probably fit (as raw data) on a single sheet of paper, but it will take a few pages more to explain what it means. First, in the 1530s, one of the Spaniards led by Cortés, upon being rewarded for his efforts with a gift of forced indigenous labor, set his forced laborers to planting Spanish hemp in the highlands around Mexico City. In 1587, a Spaniard of Atlixco, Puebla, also in the Central Highlands, requested the use of six Indians to plant hemp. It is not known whether the request was granted. About a century later, a different family, also from Atlixco, began producing hemp commercially, on a modest scale, and continued until 1761. In the 1770s, the Spanish Crown launched a concerted campaign to foment hemp production in Mexico, with indifferent success. One of the biggest problems was lack of seeds, which, according to colonial authorities, could not be bought in Mexico. And that is the entire known history of marijuana in Mexico up to that point: a few early crops of hemp, alcohol and tobacco aplenty, but no marijuana at all, strictly speaking—that is, not a word about any psychoactive cannabis.

No word, that is, were it not for a studious priest of the Central Highlands, José Antonio Alzate y Ramírez, a relative of the great Mexican poet and intellectual Sor Juana Inés de la Cruz. One day in the 1760s, Alzate y Ramírez had learned that indigenous people of his locality not far from Mexico City were consuming preparations that they called (in the native language) *pipiltzintzintlis*, concoctions that gave them access, somehow, to the spirit world. Fearing pagan idolatry, the priest acquired a bit of the mysterious pipiltzintzintlis and found to his amazement that, as far as he could see, it was simply the leaves and seeds of European cannabis. He planted a seed and what sprouted, *Cannabis sativa*, confirmed his hypothesis. It seems that, although commercial hemp production hardly existed in colonial Mexico, people, especially indigenous people, had continued to cultivate it, but, clearly, to use it for something other than fiber. Alzate y Ramírez informed those trying to grow cordage and sails for the Spanish Empire where they could find hemp seeds in Mexico. Go to the marketplace and ask for pipiltzintzintlis. Look for the indigenous *herbolarias*.

Herbolarias, herb dealers, sold bundles of dried this and that, leaves, seeds, roots, and flowers of all descriptions. A little chamomile tea, some flax seed, or a dose of psilocybin. Herbolarias were generally indigenous women, and they possessed indigenous, as well as Spanish, botanical and medicinal lore. They also knew about hallucinogens, we would say today, because Mexico has the richest hallucinogenic flora in the world, teonanácatl (mushrooms from which psilocybin is refined) and peyote (cactus buds from which mescaline is refined) being merely the best known. Religious specialists among the indigenous people had used psychoactive substances for many centuries before the Spanish came, which is one reason why the Catholic Church condemned their use as idolatrous. Pipiltzintzintlis, peyote, and teonanácatl represented the competition, so to speak—a religious experience outside the Church. Therefore, Mexico's spiritual users of cannabis kept a low profile, but the evidence of their activities was not hard to find if one knew where to look. Seeds for pipiltzintzintlis? Why didn't you say so? By the bushel!

What had happened? Without more detailed evidence, we have only inference to guide us. Apparently, during the two and a half centuries between the 1530s and the 1780s, when commercial hemp production was fizzling totally and only a handful of documents confirm its existence in Mexico, there nonetheless had been continuous subsistence cultivation of *Cannabis sativa*, a few plants here and there in rural kitchen gardens, just as in Spain or New England. It seems a safe inference. Then, let us recall that Mexico's majority rural population of these years was strongly indigenous, not Spanish landlords, for the most part, but Spanish-speaking Indians, ruled over by Spanish viceroys and bishops, but heirs to a millenarian tradition of selective cultivation. Mexico is one of the world's true hot spots of plant domestication. Corn, a Mexican creation, and, like cannabis, a wind-pollinated crop that requires constant, ongoing selection by traditional farmers, is a prime example. Domestic corn, far more than Old World grains like wheat and barley, constitutes a triumph of early bio-engineering, entirely transformed from its wild progenitors. Let us recall, next, that these botanical wizards also had a special interest in, and long experience with, hallucinogenic flora that gave privileged access to the spirit world. Anthropologists believe that the New World has so many more known hallucinogens than the Old, roughly ten times as many, not because it was providentially endowed with more, but because New World people were better at identifying them. They gained this ability, hypothetically, by migrating through so many distinct climate zones to populate the Americas. Perhaps, in view of all this, we should not be at all surprised if ten generations of indigenous Mexican botanists, aided by the blistering tropical sun, were able to discover and cultivate the psychoactive potential in European hemp.

Such, apparently, was the origin of the marijuana that eventually traveled to the United States around 1900, but we can't be certain. Perhaps the Spanish hempseeds that first arrived in Mexico had already been crossed, somehow, with *Cannabis indica* from Morocco. The Moors, Muslims gave their name to Morocco, had lived in Spain for centuries, and definitely grew psychoactive cannabis. Wind-born cannabis pollen can fly across the Strait of Gibraltar from Morocco to Spain. No Moors came to the New World, though. The indigenous people would still have had to discover the plant's psychoactive powers for themselves. Perhaps an African slave, accompanying the Spanish invasion of the New World, somehow brought a few seeds of a potent psychoactive strain with him. That seems more likely to have occurred in Brazil, where African slaves were more numerous. In any case, indigenous Mexicans, with their pipiltzintzintlis, clearly had a special role in recognizing and cultivating the plant that became marijuana.

Oddly, Alzate y Ramírez's discovery that pipiltzintzintlis exactly resembled hemp was soon forgotten, and references to pipiltzintzintlis disappeared after a few years, anyway. The low profile, again. Not until the 1840s does one find any further evidence that marijuana existed in Mexico. And then, there it is. In 1846, the recently founded Mexican Academy of Pharmacy published a national pharmacopeia that registered the existence of two separate Mexican strains of cannabis: *sativa*, listed for its "emulsive seed" (for hempseed oil, the classic, nonpsychoactive European medical use) and, in a separate entry, "Rosa María," which it also called "*native* hemp," used for its "narcotic leaves." Another name for Rosa María, according to the book, was *mariguana*, the first appearance of any form of that word in print. In the next decade, a pharmacist of the University of Guadalajara mentioned that Rosa María was smoked in cigarettes, the first evidence of that practice. (Pipiltzintzintlis seem to have been eaten.) Further references followed in the 1860s and 1870s, as the word *marihuana* gradually became familiar to readers of Mexican newspapers.

Marijuana was very far from being a universal of Mexican life, however. Little known in the cities before 1850, it grew widely in the countryside, and the smokers of it were poor country people, and not just the indigenous people whose grandparents had spoken of, and perhaps used, pipiltzintzintlis. In the 1840s and 1850s, those who spoke of and used Rosa María, which is to say marijuana, included many who had left an indigenous identity behind. Marijuana use was emerging now among mestizos, people in the not-Indian, not-European category of cultural/racial in-betweenness by which Mexicans increasingly defined their national sense of self. Undoubtedly, though not illegal, smoking Rosa María was considered un-Catholic. The oh-so-innocent-sounding name was itself a reminder of the need to blow some smoke, so to speak, when mentioning the drug. The young rural men who gathered to pass a marijuana cigarette from hand to hand were not doing anything religious, not divining the future or gaining access to the spirit world. They were using marijuana more as a cheap substitute (or enhancement) for pulque, with the difference that it did not interfere with physical labor. And yet, the idea that marijuana was a "devil weed" (as the Inquisition had considered pipiltzintzintlis to be), the idea that it was a bit pagan, that it produced madness and unholy violence—had not completely vanished, either.

Beginning in the 1860s, national upheaval and war, then a period of rapid economic growth, stirred things up in rural Mexico, moving soldiers and workers around the country. First there was the French invasion that created an imperial throne for Emperor Maximilian (under French control). Then the great hero of the Mexican resistance against the French, Porfirio Díaz, inaugurated a thirty-year period of dictatorial presidency that put out a welcome mat for international investment and enterprise. Railroad-building opened the countryside and gave it access to the Atlantic economy. That was a boon to landowners, but it tended to displace the landless peasantry. Many became hacienda "peons," which was about as nice as it sounds. Railroads offered a ride elsewhere. On the way, migrants passed through growing towns. They were young men with zero years of schooling, jostled loose from tiny, traditional villages, now far from home, willing to try their hands at anything. They landed in the army, in labor camps, in rough neighborhoods where homeless drifters go to spend the night. Often, they got in trouble for fighting. It was a commonplace belief in Mexico that *marihuana* (like pulque and tequila) made them do it.

Prisons and military barracks were the two places most associated with marijuana smoking in Mexico by 1900. We should be clear about what that means. Marijuana had not turned these conscripts into soldiers, obviously, and, consumption of it not being generally illegal, neither had it turned them into prisoners. Rather, prisons and barracks created the ideal conditions for marijuana to substitute for pulque. Mexican prisons concentrated on keeping inmates inside, not on supervising their activities there. Barracks, too, were somewhat prisonlike. Compared with alcoholic drinks, marijuana was much more easily smuggled and consumed. Prisons and barracks were also places of tough masculine society where the "devil weed" reputation could even be a plus. So "prisoner" and "soldier" make sense as far and away the most frequently mentioned identities of early marijuana users in the Mexican press. Other descriptors often applied in print were *lower class, degenerate, thieves, Indians, social dregs, police* (recruited from the social dregs), and *revolutionaries*—along with various references to women, such as *herbolarias, prostitutes,* and *soldaderas.* The denizens of Mexico City's underworld were said to loiter at cheap cafés smoking grifos and drinking coffee laced with cane liquor. Finally, there were also some middle-class dandies who dabbled in marijuana. Such a figure was drawn by the famous late-nineteenth-century caricaturist José Guadalupe Posada, who called his creation "Chepito Marihuano." A group of young dandies was said to meet at night in the shadowy cloisters of an abandoned convent, decorated with symbols of occult spiritualism, to smoke marijuana and read poetry.

Some women smoked marijuana, but press reports provide good evidence that men outnumbered them twenty to one. Women appear in the press reports much more often as suppliers than users. Herbolarias were not supposed to sell marijuana, but they remained the chief source of it for the urban population. Soldaderas, who traveled with soldiers to cook for them and take care of them in various ways, could be described as prostitutes or as soldiers' sweethearts, overlapping categories at the time. Getting marijuana from the herbolaria and sneaking it to her man in a jail or a prisonlike barracks was a routine chore for such a woman, who may never have smoked it herself.

Mexican press accounts from the late 1800s and the turn of the twentieth century present marijuana as a substance that converts smokers into homicidal maniacs after exactly three puffs. Here, in article after article, we find the origins of the "reefer madness" image later publicized in the United States by Anslinger's Federal Bureau of Narcotics. It is an open question how much this "social script" influenced the behavior of the young men who were smoking marijuana in Mexico more than a hundred years ago. Did they feel themselves possessed by a devilish influence that made (or allowed) them to run amok? Press descriptions of fights under the influence of marijuana don't differ much, in fact, from descriptions of similar fights under the influence of drink. Mentions of alcohol in such accounts were twenty to a hundred times more common. And yet, the Mexican press had absolutely nothing good to say about marijuana, whereas alcohol was a different, more complex story.

Alcohol was the active ingredient of lower-class pulque, but also of champagne and cognac, symbols of European chic in a country whose better-off citizens yearned for Europe. Only a smattering of bohemian middle-class Mexicans dabbled with marijuana, but all social classes drank. Immigrant families of German brewers were beginning to produce excellent beer in Mexico. Consequently, grisly murders, described with lurid detail in the yellow press (newspapers sometimes called, in Spanish, *prensa roja* for the color of blood, their prime subject matter), could not define the entire social meaning of alcohol, only its lowlife pathology, for the Mexican reading public of 1900. But they could, and did, define the entire meaning of marijuana. And marijuana's indigenous image only made matters more embarrassing for the Mexican middle class, by reminding them of a Mexico that they preferred to forget.

All this gives us a much better picture of the backstory, so to speak, of marijuana smoking in the United States. The U.S.-built railroads that were stirring up the Mexican countryside also hired many Mexican workers and carried them north to the U.S. border.

U.S. mining and ranching interests in northern Mexico wanted more strong young men with zero years of schooling (jostled loose from tiny villages, willing to try their hands at anything), and soon U.S. labor contractors were signing them up to repair track or pick peaches north of the border. Nobody but the young men knew they smoked marijuana, until they got into fights . . . and the rest is history, or, at least, a story already told in chapter 2. Now we can understand why Pancho Villa's soldiers sang about marijuana, why migrating workers kept the stuff under wraps, and why respectable Mexican Americans had not the slightest interest in defending it. Finally, we can see where Harry Anslinger got the idea of promoting the Marihuana Tax Act of 1937 by showing congressmen pictures of mangled corpses.

If indigenous Mexicans managed to detect and cultivate the psychoactive powers that *Cannabis sativa* had lacked in Europe, did the same thing happen elsewhere in the Americas?

COLOMBIA AND JAMAICA

The short answer is probably not. Most Latin American countries had no discernable tradition of marijuana use at all before the phenomenon was introduced from the outside in the twentieth century. Colombia is fairly typical in that regard.

Like most other Latin American countries, Colombia has only a very brief history of use—less, in fact, than the United States. If the United States learned to smoke marijuana from Mexico, a crude but accurate description, Colombia learned to smoke it from the United States. Reports from 1607, 1610, 1632, and 1789 indicate that repeated attempts to stimulate hemp production for sails and cordage had conspicuously failed in Colombia, just as happened in most of Spain's American territories, seemingly because of the deeply rooted native fiber crops, such as *fique* and *henequen*. The most successful hemp plantations were in Chile, and there is no record of any psychoactive use surrounding them.

Whatever hemp grew in Colombia, nobody smoked it, either. Then, in the mid-1920s, people began to bring marijuana to Colombia from abroad. The first mention of the drug in Colombian newspapers crops up only in the mid-1920s, on the country's Caribbean coast, around its busiest port, Barranquilla. It was apparently brought by sailors and by men who came to work on banana plantations belonging to one of the first U.S. multinationals, the United Fruit Company. You could buy it around Barranquilla at stands selling food, beer, and *guarapo*, the local fermented drink. The earliest producing areas in Colombia were in the vicinity of the United Fruit banana plantations, which probably indicates that the workers were smoking marijuana—except that it wasn't exactly *marijuana*, that is, the somewhat mysterious psychoactive strain that had appeared in Mexico. It was probably *ganja, Cannabis indica* from Jamaica. Ordinary Colombians called it by an African word, *marimba*.

From the 1890s to the 1920s, black workers of the English-speaking Caribbean (Jamaica, Trinidad, Guyana) circulated widely and often smoked marijuana, or ganja, or marimba, by whatever name. They had gotten it from East Indian laborers brought to the Caribbean by the British. The Caribbean was trade rich and labor-hungry during those years, a vortex of circulating people and goods linked to the Atlantic economy. The workers who dug the Panama Canal, that enormously labor-intensive early-twentieth-century project, came from the black Caribbean. A mobile black Caribbean workforce manned the banana plantations of Central America and Colombia. Banana plantations were connected to the "modern" world by the fast steam transportation necessary to move their fragile, perishable product to market in the United States. Bustling Barranquilla was a more modern, cosmopolitan city, in some ways, than the Colombian capital, Bogotá. In Colombia, therefore, marimba embodied "globalizing forces" in the Atlantic economy, the increasing movement of capital, commodities, and labor. As in Mexico, it was a poor man's drug (but not, in Colombia, a "devil weed").

Marimba smoking increased slightly in the 1930s and 1940s, but in general, domestic consumption has been quite secondary, in Colombia, to the illegal traffic, which only began in the 1960s, responding to the demand of the U.S. market. The tradition that launched Colombia into its "marimba bonanza" of the 1970s was not a tradition of use or cultivation. It was a tradition of smuggling, which people of the Guajira Peninsula of Colombia's Caribbean coast have carried on for hundreds of years. U.S. hippies and Colombian youth back from a brush with the U.S. counterculture ventured into the Sierra Nevada mountains behind the city of Santa Marta (not so far from the old United Fruit banana plantations), identified the quality of the product, tested the market, and began to smuggle it in personal luggage. Businessmen who had been smuggling coffee (to avoid paying export tax) saw a much more profitable opportunity, planted marimba, and began to send boatloads to the United States.

From that limited trade, in coming decades, sprang Colombia's drug cartels, their ostentatious style of spending and violence, their widening presence in national life. Beginning on the Caribbean coast, where the smugglers themselves were sometimes Guajiro Indians, the bankrollers of the operation were often businessmen from the coffee-producing central cordillera of Colombia, particularly Medellín. This part of Colombia has a reputation for entrepreneurial aggressiveness and Catholic piety, two qualities certainly on display in the drug mafia that came to be called the Medellín cartel. Colombia's decades-long experience with rural-guerrillas-cum-bandits had already begun in the 1950s and 1960s, and in the central cordillera the government often did not rule, creating myriad opportunities for illegal activities in the cordillera's steep and labyrinthine flanks.

Marimba cultivation on the Caribbean coast was upstaged in the 1980s by cocaine smuggling, centered in Medellín. At first the cocaine came from further south, from Bolivia and Peru, but soon the Medellín cartel was processing coca leaves (the raw material) in Colombia. The fabulously powerful crime boss Pablo Escobar became the most famous Colombian in the world. He and his associates purchased political influence and laundered obscene profits, driving urban real estate prices skyward. Then Colombia's rural guerrillas, who in the 1980s and 1990s controlled much of the countryside, began to finance themselves partly by "taxing" the traffic and occasionally kidnapping the narcos for ransom. The narcos resisted "taxation" by creating paramilitary forces to protect themselves against guerrilla extortion, but the paramilitaries, too, got involved in the traffic. More drug money, more gasoline on the flames. As bullets ripped through rural communities, country people caught in the crossfire fled to the major cities. When they were miffed, Colombian mafia dons like Escobar assassinated judges and detonated bombs on the streets of major cities. Not mafia ruthlessness, but rather, explosive profitability, was what made the illegal traffic unstoppable. Colombia's ruling class hated it, but, even more, they wanted a piece of it. At one point, they let Escobar design his own boutique prison just for himself and run his syndicate by cell phone. Like the rural guerrillas and the right-wing paramilitaries, the drug mafia became a fact of Colombian life, something that middle-class people simply worked around in planning their daily business and pleasure.

They also learned to consume marimba and various forms of cocaine. Marimba first became common among people of the Caribbean coast, then followed the inland expansion of the traffic. Those involved in the traffic had an abundance of marimba on hand. Middle-class kids got the message by listening to rock music. But most young Colombians were not involved in the traffic and not middle-class. They were too busy (dreaming of a car and a decent job) to "turn on, tune in, and drop out." Overall, Colombians continued to prefer beer and the cane liquor called *aguardiente* to marijuana. The annual prevalence of marijuana use in Colombia never approached the U.S. rate. It is the U.S. market, not internal consumption, that has defined the Colombian experience with cannabis.

The Jamaican experience has been different. Some rural communities of Jamaica have strong, pre–twentieth-century patterns of psychoactive cannabis use. The Jamaican word *ganja* is from Hindi, and there is little mystery about how the plant got to Jamaica. Both the word and the plant were apparently brought to Jamaica by indentured laborers from India during the nineteenth century. These men from South Asia were intended to substitute for the freed slaves of Jamaica, who, after abolition in the 1830s, refused to stay on coastal sugar plantations. Casting about for alternative labor, the British decided to import manpower under long-term contract from their vast South Asian colony. The indentured laborers, mostly Hindi speakers, earned less than the freed slaves, but they kept coming in a slow, steady stream until the 1910s. Among the things that they brought with them, in addition to the ganja itself and distinctive clothing and golden bangles, was a cylindrical ganja-smoking pipe called a *chillum*, the custom of consuming cannabis in a chilled beverage, and the propensity to think of it in religious terms.

Meanwhile, the freed slaves who preferred not to do plantation labor at any price migrated to the Jamaican highlands where they could grow their own food, and, eventually, their own ganja, too. They were following in the footsteps of escaped slaves who had made free lives for themselves there in earlier times. Maroons, they were called. By 1913, ganja was evidently well-enough established in such communities for the British colonial government to ban it. A few more years and black Jamaicans had become the primary consuming population in the country. What we know about their use of ganja comes mostly from the work of anthropologists who studied rural Jamaica in the 1970s. These anthropologists found ganja integrated into the working and social lives of rural men, most of whom smoked it, and many of whom grew their own. They used it for diversion and relaxation, but also for endurance in physical labor, and in a religious manner.

While that last inclination is plainly Indian, the Jamaican religion didn't come with the ganja. Rather, it came from the Bible, which the slaves and escaped slaves and freed slaves interpreted creatively. The Christian story of deliverance and redemption spoke to them, and they embraced it and added to it. One of the additions was ganja, which they believed opened their minds for spiritual communion. They found biblical quotations to legitimate their vision (as in Psalm 104, "He causeth the grass for the cattle, and herb for the service of man"), and came to envision themselves as heirs of the ancient Children of Israel in their Babylonian captivity. Their unusual clarity, in that regard, came from the earlier activities of Marcus Garvey, a Jamaican who claimed maroon descent and dreamed of mobilizing millions of people scattered throughout the African

diaspora in the Americas. During the 1920s, Garvey had created quite a stir with his "Pan-Africanist" activities in several parts of the Atlantic world, his founding of a Universal Negro Improvement Association and an African Communities League, and his creation of the Black Star Shipping Line, as well as his exhortations to self-help and cooperation among people of African descent around the world. Garvey predicted that a great leader would arise in Africa to head the movement. Some saw the 1930 crowning of Ethiopia's emperor Haile Selassie as the rise of that leader. Wishful thinking. But faith does not require evidence, and even though the emperor of Ethiopia (Ras Tafari, he was called, before ascending his throne as Haile Selassie) never did anything to redeem the modern Children of Israel who yearned for deliverance and redemption and smoked ganja in their search for it, he did furnish them a name: Rastafarians. And he did visit Jamaica, in 1966, so the devotion of the island's Rastafarians had at least not passed unnoticed by him.

Among those inspired by the emperor's visit was a young musician, Bob Marley, who brought Rastafarianism to the attention of the world. Marley was an exponent of the musical style known as reggae, a supremely diasporic mixture of influences, and his international concert tours of the 1970s made reggae an enduring part of the world music scene. Marley's long hair (his "dreadlocks"), which Rastafarians are not supposed to cut, and his unapologetic ganja smoking put him right in stride with other popular musicians of the period, such as the Rolling Stones and the Grateful Dead. Like them, he was arrested repeatedly.

Marley was not a Jamaican expression of the U.S. counterculture, but rather something more homegrown, an authentically popular Jamaican voice, who represented a style of cannabis use that owed nothing to Haight-Ashbury. What was new for Jamaica, in 1968, was not long hair and cannabis but the surging market for Jamaican ganja in Woodstock Nation. Whereas little evidence of Jamaican ganja in the United States occurs before that point, given its notable potency and the proximity of Jamaica to the United States, an illegal trade grew rapidly in the 1970s and 1980s. As in Colombia, the drug traffic eventually represented a sizeable portion of Jamaica's gross national product.

In the 1970s, Colombia and Jamaica had begun to export *indica* strains of marijuana that were much stronger than the Mexican variety and that retailed in the United States for three times as much. The Colombian and Jamaican experiences converge most notably in the disastrous impact of that traffic on national life. But the contrasts between these two cases are more meaningful than the similarities. Jamaica's marijuana culture represents a direct connection with India, something unique in the hemisphere. Aside from those already discussed, only one other Latin American country had marijuana smokers before the United States did: Brazil.

BRAZIL AND THE AFRICAN CONNECTION

Brazil's tradition remains relatively unstudied, which seems a bit odd. Today, marijuana is exuberantly present among urban youth, rich and poor, a fixture, particularly, of the improvised neighborhoods called *favelas*, and so it's been for decades. Before the 1960s, however, things were quite different.

Brazilians may have been the first to smoke marijuana in the New World, and the story, once again, seems to involve a migration of laborers, in this case, the involuntary migration of enslaved Africans. In Jamaica, Colombia, and the United States, as we have seen, people of African descent figured significantly among smokers of cannabis at some point in the twentieth century. In none of those cases, however, do the slaves appear to have brought it with them from Africa. Brazilian *maconha*, on the other hand, seems to have a direct African origin. For example, Brazilians call it by a variety of African names, and they once smoked it in water pipes of a distinctively African design.

In describing the creation of the Atlantic World in the 1500s, we mentioned the huge part played by sugar. Let's now consider the slave labor that cultivated, harvested, and milled the sugarcane. The two great centers of sugar production for Atlantic trade were Brazil and the Caribbean, equally characterized by their reliance on enslaved African labor. Brazil was the first great sugar producer of the Americas and, as such, became the greatest single destination

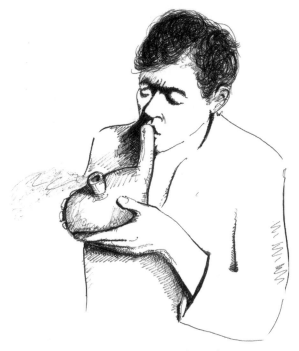

A Brazilian water pipe of African design.

of the slave trade. Rather than being truly a "single destination," though, colonial Brazil was a string of Portuguese settlements that hardly communicated with one another. They had one big thing in common, their dependency on slave labor, beginning in the 1500s. Slavery saturated Brazil, no corner of society was free of it, and it lasted for three hundred years. Because Brazil juts far east into the South Atlantic, it is much nearer to Africa than is the United States. That made slaves less costly, so more were imported, and slavery became ubiquitous in Brazilian life. In Brazil, even freed slaves sometimes owned slaves. It was an exceptional but well-known phenomenon. So old João has bought a slave of his own, has he? Eyebrows go up. He must be doing well! Brazilian slavery was not totally abolished until 1888.

There is a clear consensus, among the few who have considered the matter, that slaves brought maconha to Brazil. It makes sense. Brazil's close connection to Africa allowed for the transatlantic transfer of African foods, clothing styles, and religious practices—importations that Brazilians celebrate as aspects of the nation's cultural heritage. Furthermore, when a few Brazilians began to study maconha in the early twentieth century, they found it most often among people of African descent. In sum, the idea of maconha's deep roots in the long experience of slavery is persuasive and probably correct. The caveat, for this global history, is a troubling lack of direct evidence.

Like Mexican marijuana, Brazilian maconha is practically invisible in the historical record until the late nineteenth century, partly because Brazilians were busy consuming other drugs instead. Abundant sugar made Brazilian cane liquor (called *cachaça*) also abundant. Mixed with further sugar and lime juice, it became the national drink, practically replacing milder, fermented drinks until the twentieth century. As in Mexico and the United States, the indigenous drug of choice, tobacco, flourished in colonial Brazil, too. Cachaça and tobacco were both useful in the slave trade, as well as for domestic consumption. These drugs were widely (and intensively) ingested by Portuguese settlers, their descendants, and pretty much everybody else in Brazil, too. Maconha, on the other hand, was used primarily by plantation slaves and other poor rural people, who wrote nothing about it, being the least literate group in society. Plantation owners (another group that wrote little) appear to have tolerated it. Anthropologist Gilberto Freyre, the influential nationalist interpreter of Brazil's African heritage, wrote in the 1930s that earlier plantation owners had allowed slaves to cultivate maconha between the rows of sugarcane. Freyre knew a great deal about Brazilian slavery, both from his research in historical sources and from his plantation-family background, but he gave no evidence for his assertion. In fact, aside from a handful of anecdotes, the chief evidence for Brazilian maconha's African origins is a series of central African names that Brazilians used for it in the late nineteenth and early twentieth centuries, *maconha* being only the best known. In the 1940s and before, *diamba* was more common, and another term was *fumo de Angola*, which could be translated as "Angolan tobacco." However, none of those names occur in writing before the twentieth century. And then there's the "old saying" of the slave masters that "smoking maconha makes the blacks lazy," which was not recorded before the twentieth century, either.

So, stepping back from the pervasive but vague oral tradition, what proof exists of maconha's presence in Brazil before the twentieth century? The first contemporary trace of maconha in Brazil (potentially, anyway) occurs in a legal document dated 1747. The "crime" in question isn't quite clear. Inquisitors were interrogating a young man accused of illicit sexual activities (with other young men), when he admitted that they had gotten "loaded" by drinking and smoking before their frolic. He didn't say what they had been smoking, and the inquisitors didn't ask. They were more focused on the sex. Interestingly, this young man was a musician from Portugal, although his buddies were partly of African descent. A second contemporary trace (presuming that it is accurate) comes only in 1830, when the city council of Rio de Janeiro supposedly banned the sale of *pito de pango*, a name for maconha on the East African coast. The document is widely mentioned but is not preserved in any archive. Then, in 1867, an English traveler described slaves frittering away their Sundays smoking what he termed "hashish," which he had also encountered in India and on the African coast. There are a few other random anecdotes, a weak form of historical evidence.

This is alarmingly little documentation for a supposedly widespread activity over a period of centuries. True enough, the shreds of evidence that we do have—legal prohibitions, judicial inquiries, and travelers' accounts—*are* commonly the historical glimpses that one gets of cultural activities scorned by the Brazilian ruling class. In conjunction with oral traditions, they confirm that maconha *was* present in Brazil by the mid-1800s. But they give no reliable indication of how, or from where, maconha *came to* Brazil. After all, African words might just as naturally have been applied by Africans to a familiar-looking plant (Portuguese hemp) that Europeans had definitely planted in Brazil. In fact, the notable lack of written evidence, despite decades of slavery studies, shows that maconha simply cannot have been very common among slaves, in Brazil or anywhere else in the New World. Police, travelers, and plantation owners would have left more written evidence about a common practice. Instead, maconha emerges in Brazilian history, much as marijuana emerges in Mexican history, from rustic anonymity to urban notoriety, only toward the beginning of the twentieth century.

When Brazilian public health officials finally began to study maconha in the mid-twentieth century, they identified it as a regional phenomenon, an aspect of *northern* Brazil, relatively unknown in the south. Their explanation was climate, the more intense sun of the equatorial north. Interestingly, the areas of intense plantation agriculture, Brazil's demographic black belts, created by sugar and coffee cultivation, mostly along the coast, were *not* the rural roots identified by twentieth-century officials diagnosing the maconha problem. Rather, they indicated the backlands, the fringe areas of original Portuguese settlement in the arid northern interior, the sorts of places still inhabited by catechized Indians, places where the descendants of African slaves were a minority. The idea is suggestive.

Public health officials of the mid-twentieth century associated maconha with people of indigenous descent, as well as blacks, listing *fumo de caboclo*, which could be translated as "Indian tobacco," as one of its slang appellatives, along with *fumo de Angola*. Might Brazil's indigenous peoples have discerned and developed European hemp's latent psychoactive potential, as seems to have occurred in Mexico? Anthropologists have identified maconha use among some Amazonian Indians. Although Brazil does not duplicate Mexico's profusion of hallucinogenic flora, the native Amazonian drug *ayahuasca* (an ingenious combination of two different plants) shows an obvious alertness to the potential of such flora. Successful selective cultivation of European hemp to encourage its psychoactive properties would have taken time, as in Mexico, and it would have occurred away from prying Portuguese eyes, in the indigenous backlands. It would probably have had some kind of spiritual application, similar to whatever it was people did with pipiltzintzintlis in Mexico. It would have been disseminated slowly, by contact and migration, and spread first from Indians to blacks and mestizo peasants, those least able to afford tobacco and cachaça. This is, in fact, the pattern we can dimly see in the evidence. A native Brazilian "invention" of maconha, similar to the native Mexican "invention" of marijuana, just might have occurred. For now, though, the brought-from-Africa scenario seems more probable for Brazil.

Fortunately, the history of maconha becomes clearer in the mid-twentieth century. It looks much like the early history of marijuana. Evidence shows that the smokers of maconha lived mostly in the north, were mostly black, most often male, invariably poor and downtrodden. This was a period of rural-to-urban migration, and people who smoked maconha were often new to the city. Inevitably, they were marginal, too. Street children were especially known for maconha. As in Mexico, barracks and prisons (also mental hospitals and brothels) were common places to find smokers. So were ports, right at the waterfront; fishermen and other boatmen sometimes kept a water pipe in their boats. The São Francisco River, the great transportation artery of the Brazilian backlands, was the central axis of maconha production and distribution. The river-port town of Propiá in the state of Sergipe had a particular reputation for the quality of its product, which was distributed by boat up and down the Atlantic coast to the waterfronts of larger cities, like Bahia and Recife. Smoking maconha, by the twentieth century, was done mostly in cigarettes rather than water pipes, often in lively groups called "assemblies" that engaged in competitive, rhyming wordplay. Local color fiction writers depicted such assemblies using invented nonsense rhymes of African-sounding words. A boy who grew up in Propiá recalled the rambunctious, entertaining late-afternoon assemblies in the marketplace there.

In the 1930s, northeastern intellectuals became interested in maconha as an expression of regional folk culture. At the same time, however, Brazil created its own Federal Bureau of Narcotics, which took an Anslinger-like stand against the maconha menace. During the 1940s, U.S. soldiers stationed in Bahia did not find maconha difficult to acquire, and Bahian public health officials became worried about the soldiers excessively stimulating the market. Still, as late as the 1950s, smoking maconha remained relatively rare in Brazil, especially in the major urban areas of the south, the principal centers of Brazilian national life. The real stimulation occurred in the

1960s and afterward, among Brazilian youth who were inspired by the international counterculture. By the mid-1980s, smoking maconha had become a sign of modernity. The U.S. market was too far away to beckon strongly, but Brazil's internal market was big enough to generate a lucrative trade, especially in urban giants like Rio de Janeiro and São Paulo. Poor neighborhoods passed under the control of gangs of twenty-something drug merchants wearing flip-flops and brandishing assault weapons.

The persuasiveness of the brought-from-Africa hypothesis for Brazilian maconha lies not in the evidence, which is sketchy, but in its overall historical logic. Around 1500, when the diaspora of African slaves began, Africa south of the Congo River was the only part of the Atlantic World where people used cannabis psychoactively.

AFRICA, SOUTH OF THE CONGO

Available evidence of early cannabis drugs in Africa is even scarcer than what we have for the Americas. But it is consistent and unambiguous regarding the area south of the Congo River. Moreover, cannabis drugs definitely circulated in the slave trade.

There exists at least one African travel account of a cannabis seed in the possession of a captive awaiting exportation. There exists at least one other in which a slave trader introduces the custom to an African associate. Like most people in the Americas, however, Africans showed a consistent and unambiguous preference for ethanol as a recreational drug.

Virtually all the societies of sub-Saharan Africa made and consumed fermented drinks. The most distinctive, also the most potent, was wine made from the sap of the raphia palm, the African analogue of Mexican pulque. It was men's work to climb the tree and tap the sweet, milky fluid that fermented very quickly in the hot climate. Palm wine had to be drunk immediately, most often in a single day. Raphia palms were widespread but limited in numbers. The alternative drink was beer made from native grains, normally a kind of millet or sorghum. Beer making, which involved sprouting the grain to malt it, then baking it, then fermenting it for several days, was much more laborious and protracted. Consequently, brewing was usually women's work, viewed as an offshoot of cooking, which beer making has most often been in traditional societies around the world. This sort of beer had a much lower alcohol content than palm wine, as low as 2 percent, but it was quite nutritious and, like most historical beer, had the consistency of gruel. Palm wine and millet beer were drunk to celebrate social gatherings, to close commercial contracts, to bond with new relations at a wedding party, to facilitate tears at a funeral, and to communicate with departed spirits. Africans showed their esteem for ethanol by reserving it mostly for their "big men," the senior leaders of villages, clans, tribes, and kingdoms. Still, though widely produced and highly valued, ethanol was less abundant in Africa than elsewhere in the Atlantic World.

The magic of altered consciousness was a scarce resource in Africa, often a perquisite of the powerful. It belonged to a more general category of scarce resource: food. Most of Africa's economies were subsistence economies, geared to produce sufficiency, with little surplus. Senior males drank deeply themselves and also distributed the prized substance to their friends and followers. Younger men, and women of any age, were less likely to consume alcohol in Africa. Few other generalizations can be made about psychoactive drugs in these extremely diverse, small-scale societies, except to say that, around 1500, cannabis, too, seems to have been present in many of them.

Cannabis was much newer and more sparsely and unevenly represented in sub-Saharan African life than was ethanol, however. Once again, only a tiny smattering of written references exists, in contrast to a much better documented history of drink. European travelers make scattered mention of cannabis, using especially the words *dagga* and *riamba*, mostly in the 1800s. A few broad outlines emerge from what they say. Above all, they indicate that Africans pioneered *smoking* cannabis. Archeological evidence now shows the existence of pipes predating the introduction of tobacco to Africa. There are a great variety of water-pipe designs, including a number made from gourds, as would later be common in Brazil. Several travelers found people smoking to prepare for war, and another found them doing it to make peace. It was used for physical work and for rest and recreation. The famous explorer Livingstone wrote that "all the tribes of the interior" used the pernicious and stupefying weed.

Nothing clearly differentiates what we know of cannabis in precolonial Africa from patterns of alcohol use there. People apparently smoked in the absence of alcohol or to augment its effect. Several illustrations from Angola in the early 1800s show men smoking water pipes while drinking. In one of those illustrations, the men are drinking, probably cachaça that was brought from Brazil to trade for slaves. Once again, the preferred euphoriant was alcohol, but the great advantage of cannabis was the ease with which it can be grown, stored, and transported, attributes making it less costly. It is indicative, surely, that the hunter-gathering Khoisan peoples, the Bushmen of Africa's southern deserts—whose material culture is totally minimalist—were early adopters of *dagga*, as they called it, applying a name formerly used for another hallucinogen, *datura*. Notably, they were not using cannabis to replace alcohol, but something much stronger.

Cannabis had been south of the Congo River for only a few hundred years when Europeans arrived. Linguistic studies indicate that it was introduced on Africa's east coast, along the shores of the Indian Ocean, sometime between the years 1000 and 1300, and then diffused gradually westward. (See map.) *Bhang*, the traditional name for cannabis on Africa's east coast, comes from Hindi. From 1000 to 1500, Indian Ocean traders plied the east coast of Africa, linking it closely to India, the core area of global cannabis culture. Most of these traders were Muslims, and Islam became the religion of Africa's east coast. The natives of that coast became cultural intermediaries whose Swahili language, combining Bantu syntax with Arabic vocabulary, served as a lingua franca. Swahili intermediaries apparently learned to use bhang from the traders and then disseminated it inland. The westward diffusion of bhang can be traced in the changing names applied to the drug. By the time it reached the shores of the Atlantic in Angola and the Congo, it was called *riamba*, and eventually *diamba*, names that turned up later in Brazil.

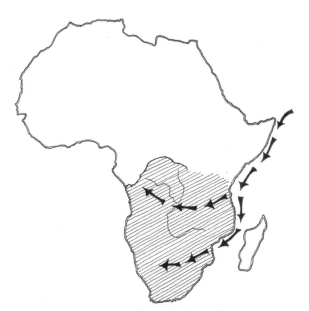

Cannabis, south of the Congo River.

Curiously, the east-to-west dissemination of psychoactive cannabis seems to have stopped at the Congo River. While the slave trade probably introduced it at a few points on the West African coast, West African societies overall lack traditional names for psychoactive cannabis and have tended to adopt international ones, such as "weed." This picture substantiates the notion of east-to-west diffusion, obviously, but it constitutes a mystery, as well, given the existence of trans-Saharan communications and the importance of hashish in Mediterranean Africa after about 1000, as will be discussed later. For now, we will focus on the southern region where cannabis clearly *was* present by the 1600s.

On Africa's Swahili coast, bhang had the prestige of an exotic trade good, associated with fine cities like Kilwa, the impressive port admired by the world traveler Ibn Battuta in the 1300s. Bhang probably began its westward journey on caravans connecting the coast to gold-producing areas inland, the early states of Great Zimbabwe and Mutapa. Moving south under the name *dagga*, the drug's use was extended across the current territory of South Africa some time before 1652, when the Dutch established Cape

Town as a halfway provisioning station for Dutch ships on the way to Asia. The Khoisan people's taste for dagga led the Dutch to offer it to their laborers as a fringe benefit. The nearby Zulus, renowned warriors, figure among the people known to have used marijuana for war, but that was not until the 1800s.

As bhang moved west from the Swahili coast across central Africa, adopting the modified name *riamba*, it entered a kind of war zone. A substantial Portuguese presence created the continent's most invasive slave trade on the Atlantic coast south of the Congo River. The Portuguese introduced goods, including both guns and Brazilian cachaça, which were carried by caravan to slave fairs deep in the interior, fueling conflict. Armed conflict always disrupts food production, and ethanol is food. Cutting down raphia palms was a common act of war in Africa. A reduction of the food supply encouraged people to substitute riamba for beer. In addition, the slave traders and their associates spread various drugs around, sometimes including riamba, no doubt. As for alcohol and tobacco, they were basic to the trade. Luanda, the Portuguese import-export depot on the Atlantic coast, was full of cachaça and taverns in the 1600s and 1700s, so the big men with slaves to trade along the caravan routes were well supplied with spirits. Their followers, too, got at least a symbolic taste of cachaça. Overall, however, the toll taken by slaving probably reduced the supply of traditional fermented intoxicants among the less prosperous and encouraged the adoption of riamba.

The Beni Riamba, a short-lived "riamba brotherhood" that formed in central Africa in the 1850s (when the slave trade had finally ended) suggests further possibilities. According to a European traveler who happened to record this phenomenon, it occurred among a people known as the Bashilange, who had the sort of small-scale social organization more common in African history than large kingdoms. The numerous Bashilange clans and villages had traditionally feuded among themselves until a young leader arose proposing a new, more peaceful order against the resistance of change-averse elders. He did so, it would appear, by mobilizing an "age set," a distinctive facet of African social organization that brings together generations across clan, tribal, or ethnic dividing lines. The vehicle of peace was to be riamba.

To bring about their brotherhood, the young men smoked together in the evenings and employed riamba to settle disputes and for ritual functions. The Beni Riamba stopped inter-village feuding, making the Bashilange more industrious and prosperous. All this is according to the single traveler's account, which unfortunately is the only one we have. Still, one would not suspect a European traveler of exaggerating the benefits of "riamba brotherhood." The innovation remained localized, though, provoking a traditionalist opposition from the elders, and the Beni Riamba disappeared forever in the 1870s.

Cannabis use has certainly increased in Africa over the intervening century-plus. For one thing, it is now quite present in West Africa, especially Nigeria, the continent's most populous country. Rural users in South Africa long preferred the traditional water pipe, but urban people smoke cigarettes. This is probably true of twenty-first-century African users in general. Aside from a major sociological study of 1970s South Africa, few other primary sources of information exist. Data collected by the UN in the first decade of the twenty-first century remain sketchy, with many countries unrepresented. Regarding the number of consumers, there is a yawning gap between high estimates and low ones. High estimates put annual prevalence of marijuana use in Africa around U.S. levels—which is to say, among the highest in the world—10 percent of the population, whereas low estimates are less than half that. Zambia, a central African country with strong traditions of historical use, stands out as a hot spot in the UN data, along with Nigeria. Even more than the history of marijuana in Latin America, though, the history of marijuana in Africa largely remains to be written.

A global history of marijuana is limited at every turn, it seems, by a dearth of reliable evidence. What sound generalizations can be made about cannabis in the Atlantic World? First, we have seen its crucial importance as a European fiber crop, linked above all to maritime applications. European colonists introduced hemp practically everywhere they went in the Americas. Second, we have seen marijuana constantly overshadowed by alcohol as a recreational euphoriant. Latin American traditions of cannabis drugs are far more limited than many people imagine. Only Mexico, Jamaica, and Brazil had significant local traditions before the international influence of the U.S. counterculture made marijuana stylish in the late 1960s. While widespread in central and southern Africa before European colonization, psychoactive cannabis was nonetheless a relatively recent arrival there, too. Despite the striking account of the Beni Riamba brotherhood, most historical African societies seem to have used psychoactive cannabis much as they used alcohol. That is, much as Europeans used alcohol, although in smaller quantities. Until the 1960s, marijuana was mostly a poor man's recreational drug, not only in the United States but in the entire Atlantic World.

There are hints of something more than recreation, too: indigenous Mexican fortune tellers eating pipiltzintzintlis; Rastafarians finding ganja in the Bible; and, above all, those Beni Riamba brothers renouncing ancient feuds over peace pipes to found their brief utopia. To see the spiritual dimension of marijuana's global history more sharply delineated, we'll turn to the medieval Muslim world, which had a counterculture of its own.

4

✳

Medieval Hashish

Before the advent of marijuana, the European and U.S. experience with psychoactive cannabis came primarily from hashish. Europe's drug-dabbling avant-garde writers experimented with hashish in the mid-1800s. Harry Anslinger's 1937 portrait of the marijuana-smoker-as-homicidal-maniac explained, by way of supporting evidence, that the word *assassin* derives etymologically from *hashish*. For many centuries, in Muslim societies stretching from Spain and Morocco to Egypt, Arabia, Syria, Iraq, Iran, Afghanistan, Pakistan, and on across India to (eventually) Malaysia and Indonesia—hashish was a social fixture, though never a custom of the majority. The years 1100–1400, when hashish became established in the Muslim world, are a major chapter in our story.

First, a definition of the main term. In contemporary English, the word *hashish* refers to the pungent resin concentrated from large numbers of female cannabis flowers. During the last few centuries, certain mountainous regions of Morocco, Lebanon, Afghanistan, Pakistan, and Nepal have specialized in the production of hashish, going about it in rather different ways. In Lebanon, for example, dried cannabis flowers are rubbed through progressively finer mesh to produce a reddish powder that is then pressed into bricks.

In Nepal, for a second example, harvesters in the fields squeeze resinous flowers between their hands, accumulating layers of sticky, dark-colored hashish on their palms before scraping it off and rolling it into balls. A tiny lump of this sort of hashish produces a strong psychoactive effect. Medieval *hashish*, in contrast, was not the concentrated resin of today. Medieval hashish was described as "leafy" and must have been something like today's *sin semilla*.

Second, nobody in the Muslim world was smoking anything in the years 1100–1400. Despite the independent invention of pipe-smoking in Africa, smoking among Muslims (and as a global phenomenon) started with tobacco, and tobacco did not enter the Muslim world before the 1500s. When it did, hookahs (and other water pipes) became a common way to consume hashish, often mixed with tobacco. Before that, however, hashish was always eaten, and that requires a bit of explanation. If it is to function psychoactively in the digestive tract, marijuana must be cooked to activate its cannabinoids before eating. That is because much of the psychoactive THC exists in the raw plant as a slightly different, *non*psychoactive molecule (called THCA). Cooking above 200° F converts the THCA into THC, which happens automatically in smoking.

There were many ways to eat medieval hashish. Hashish confections involving spices, nuts, and honey were common ways to consume the plant. Another common approach was to gently roast the hashish, then roll it into little balls that could be swallowed easily. Most of the time, though, cooking with cannabis meant extracting the cannabinoids from the leaves and flowers. Cannabinoids are fat-soluble rather than water-soluble. To dissolve and extract them, you simmer the leaves and flowers in butter until it turns green, then discard the vegetable matter and cook with the infused butter.

Now that we're clear on what we are talking about, let's turn to the evidence. There are substantial written sources concerning hashish in the Arabic-speaking center of the medieval Muslim world. Interpreting them will require attention to the social and, especially, the legal and religious contexts. The crucial starting place is the status of intoxicating drink for observant Muslims.

WINE VERSUS HASHISH

The Qur'an—which Muslims regard as the direct, revealed word of God and the starting point of lawgiving—makes a clear, although somewhat complex, judgment on wine. Wine is a symbol of heavenly bounty, and the rivers of paradise run with it. But on earth wine is an impediment to Godly living. Drunkenness prevents a person from scrupulous fulfillment of earthly obligations, such as frequent prayer. In addition to the direct world of God in the Qur'an, which religious men began to commit to memory verbatim during the life of Muhammad (ca. 570–632), there accumulated a voluminous body of sacred wisdom, called *hadith*. Hadiths are traditional accounts of the Prophet's life and words, meticulously vetted by legal and religious scholars. Hadiths serve as a second tier of Muslim scripture, less authoritative and more homely than the Qur'an, and (unlike the Qur'an) evolving over time. A vast number of hadiths and commentaries on hadiths enjoin observant Muslims not to partake of alcoholic beverages. The prohibitions of wine laid down in the Qur'an and elaborated by hadith over many centuries have had a powerful cumulative impact on Islamic societies, whose limited consumption of alcohol has stood in notable contrast to the tippling customs of Christian Europe.

The Old Testament is repeatedly critical of drunkenness, but it accepts wine as an ordinary part of life and an instrument of religious ritual. In the New Testament, Jesus instructs his disciples to reenact the Last Supper using bread and wine. This reenactment, the Eucharist, became central to both Roman and Greek variants of Christianity. Because Christians needed a constant supply of wine for ritual purposes, medieval monastic orders planted their own vineyards, spreading viticulture, and a taste for the grape, throughout Europe. In addition, northern Europeans drank quite a lot of beer, or more precisely, beer and ale, the latter fermented somewhat differently. England's history of ale drinking is particularly well documented. It indicates that during the Middle Ages, the common people—men, women, and children—consumed ale daily, sometimes several times a day, including with breakfast.

This ale contained little ethanol, and it was thick, with bits of grain floating in it. In essence, ale was a way to eat barley. Fermentation served partly as a preservative. In sum, alcohol beverages constituted a basic part of the European diet, and a few extra cups more were normally available if people desired to engage in a little drunken carousing.

The Muslim repression of fermented drinks, in contrast, opened a tentative space for hashish as the-intoxicant-not-prohibited-by-the-Qur'an. Hashish was often seen as an alternative to wine. It was called "the green one" (as opposed to "the red one") in frequent poems comparing the two. However, the difference in moral status was only relative. Hashish had not yet appeared in Arabia during the life of the Prophet, so the Qur'an naturally has nothing to say about it. Its subsequent appearance in Damascus, Baghdad, and Cairo, at the center of the medieval Muslim world, brought a legal reaction against hashish. Eventually, the ongoing elaboration of hadiths included new, negative references to hashish. And, as has been explained, hadiths are quasi-scriptural in character. Some of the new criticisms were attributed directly to Muhammad, giving them more authority. For example, in one hadith, the Prophet says, "beware the green one, for it is the greatest wine," in another, "beware the wine of the Persians, for it will make you forget the confession of faith"—"the wine of the Persians," according to that hadith, being hashish. Overall, however, the prohibition against "the red one" was crystal clear, and the religious disapproval of "the green one," more debatable.

This mild-but-marked disapproval of hashish in the Sunni tradition is one key to our story. Though hardly abundant, documentation of hashish in the medieval Muslim world is better than anything we have on premodern Latin America or Africa. Moreover, much of that evidence is legal. A score of juridical treatises, in addition to hadith, have survived to illuminate the story of hashish, casting the drug in a steadily negative light. Lacking Qur'anic authority, legal scholars made alternative arguments against hashish. They reasoned that intoxication itself being the reason wine was banned, intoxicating hashish should be banned by analogy. And they further justified prohibition by enumerating harms caused by the drug, the full catalog of which is harrowing indeed:

> It destroys the mind, cuts short the reproductive capacity, produces elephantiasis, passes on leprosy . . . makes the mouth smell foul, dries up the semen, causes the eyebrows to fall out . . . causes a shortage of breath, creates strong illusions, diminishes the powers of the soul, reduces modesty, makes the complexion yellow, blackens the teeth, riddles the liver with holes, [and] inflames the stomach . . .

This example can stand for many.

Legal sources have nothing good to say about hashish. Users (normally male) were condemned as effeminate (often erotically attracted to boys) and neglectful of their religious obligations. They were out of touch with reality, debased, shiftless, and, therefore, poor. Often, hashish itself had been their ruination. Medieval Muslim jurists regarded the green one as more addictive, even, than the red one. In fact, though less lurid, the image of the hashish eater most often encountered in medieval Arabic legal sources partly resembles the figure of the modern crack or meth addict, reduced to misery because of his own improvidence, spending all his money on drugs, his very existence an affront to the idea of a well-ordered society. And the search for a well-ordered society is at the very heart of majority Sunni Islam. Disapproving legal sources were emphasized by the distinguished Yale scholar of Arabic literature Franz Rosenthal in his 1971 book, *The Herb*, which remains by far the best study of hashish in the medieval Muslim world.

Fortunately, legal sources are not the only ones to have survived. Medieval Muslim societies revered the written word and put it to various uses. An alternative and lesser known source of documentary evidence is a "bohemian" tradition of Arabic poetry, dedicated to both wine and hashish. *The Herb* contains careful translations of ten such poems, including several that compare wine to hashish and one in praise of combining them. The poems have a frankly celebratory mood that is a world away from the legal condemnations. The poetic hashish is "the wine of the poor." It is a wonderful "secret." Hashish, unlike wine grapes, has never been trodden under foot and crushed through people's toes. Nor has the green one ever been used to perform hocus-pocus at Christian altars. It is something fun and new and stylish and less sinful than wine. Anti-hashish poems, on the other hand, scoff at "the green one" as "grass" fit for beasts, while wine, on the other hand, "covers the lowly person with respectability," because of its expense. Like wine, hashish represents unearned ecstasy. Such poetry, which would have been recited at festive gatherings, provides a useful counterpoint to the dour legal treatises. A final source comprises a few medieval folk tales recounted in *One Thousand and One Nights* and elsewhere, which offer a comical view, as we will observe in a moment.

Less sinful than wine, but also less prestigious, hashish was legally condemned by the Sunni tradition, yet secretly celebrated by various sorts of fringe elements and dissenters. Before we get to the dissenters, though, let's see how the green one first appeared in Iraq, Syria, and Egypt, the center of the Muslim world, around 1100, and then discuss the use that might be called simply "recreational."

HASHISH IN MUSLIM SOCIETY

Hashish appeared in the center of the Muslim world around the year 1100, when that world was under threat. The political and religious unity of Islam, represented by the rule of a caliph in Baghdad, was dwindling away to nothing amid storms of political and religious dissent. Destructive invaders, the Crusaders of Western Europe, had entered the Muslim world from the west, and other equally alien invaders were on their way from the east. Understandably, in this context, many medieval Arabic speakers saw hashish as a harbinger of troubled times.

The first sign of hashish to appear (to those of us peering back nine hundred years) is the word itself, which occurs in Arabic-language documents beginning with one dated 1123 on the European calendar. More precisely, the 1123 document contains the first known appearance of the word *hashish* referring to a cannabis drug. The word *cannabis* (*qinnab* in Arabic) had long existed in the eastern Mediterranean, with no connection to intoxicating drugs, and the same could be said for hemp (*banj* in Arabic). As for *hashish*, it was a familiar Arabic word that, around 1123, acquired a new meaning. Before that time, *hashish* had referred vaguely to animal fodder (grass), medicinal plants (herbs), or unwanted growth in the garden (weeds). Get it? The new cannabis drug was being called "grass" or "herb" or "weed." Hashish was medieval Arabic *slang*, in other words, that eventually became the standard Arabic term for the drug.

Alias "the green one," hashish had many other aliases. A long list of them includes about seventy. Many are associated with particular regions or cities. For example, the people of Baghdad (supposedly) called hashish "the daughter of the bag," a play on the common expression "daughter of the cask" (wine). Certain professions and social types supposedly had their own code terms for hashish. Many of these terms seem fanciful inventions, but others had evident currency. Porters (supposedly) called hashish "the one that lightens the load"; philosophers, "the morsel of thought"; songstresses, "branches of bliss"—and so on, through gypsies, leather workers, cooks, water carriers, builders, homosexuals, astrologers, grave diggers, corpse washers, dealers in herbs and potions, falconers, merchants, and pimps, ending with Satan and his cohorts, who called hashish "the huntress." The "devil's own list of hashish synonyms," as it is called, critiques the wide, but normally covert, use of the drug.

Hashish was collected wild, grown in private gardens and public parks, and cultivated commercially for sale. At certain times, in certain places, it was tolerated and taxed, but the authorities occasionally cracked down on growers. There is news of crops being burned in Cairo in 1253, for example, then again in 1324. In contrast to taverns, which could exist because non-Muslims were often free to drink wine, one found no public establishments for eating hashish. Instead, there were particular streets, or houses, or shady spots where hashish eaters gathered to carouse, and perhaps recite verses in praise of the green one. Several anecdotes mention hashish eaters in the public baths that were a common feature of urban life in medieval Muslim cities. Use of intoxicants was hidden in such settings, and that went double for the center of public life, the mosque. When it came to secret recreational drug use, the green "daughter of the bag" was proverbially more portable and more easily concealed than the red "daughter of the cask."

The lower cost of hashish, when compared to wine, was also proverbial. The popularity of hashish among the urban lower classes clearly rested on its inexpensiveness. When wealthy Muslims allowed themselves to be naughty, they preferred the red one. Surely no caliph ever tasted hashish, said a poet, but many drank wine, as was well known. The average hashish eater was more like the watchman at a Cairo warehouse who supposedly spent all his wages on his habit. The religious dissidents who ate hashish, such as the followers of Haydar (to be discussed later in this chapter) did so as part of a life of poverty. The list of occupations provided by "the devil's own list of hashish synonyms" is definitely heavy on manual labor and less reputable avocations. Without a quantitative assessment of the drug's social distribution, which is plainly impossible, we can nonetheless observe clearly that Sunni jurists, whose writings have provided most of our evidence, considered hashish eaters to be the dregs of society.

Poor students were among the usual suspects. Medieval Muslim students spent many years achieving mastery over authoritative legal and religious texts. Once that mastery was achieved, moreover, it wasn't necessarily lucrative. One anecdote tells of a scholar lecturing under the influence of hashish when his turban fell off, revealing the concealed drug. Another story tells of a student who arrives unexpectedly at his teacher's home to find him deliriously dancing and reciting poetry about flowers.

Sunni jurists often accused hashish eaters of sexual deviance, especially homosexuality. They called hashish "the seducer's friend," a weapon deployed against innocent and unsuspecting targets. Popular depictions such as those in *One Thousand and One Nights* emphasize the erotic fantasies and promiscuity of hashish eaters. *One Thousand and One Nights* is a treasury of medieval folk tales from around the Muslim world, combined in a framing narrative wherein, to avoid her execution (perpetually threatened for the next day, for reasons that don't matter here) a woman, Scheherazade, must entertain the prince with her storytelling. She chooses the most compelling material—bawdy, lurid, and action-packed—and she cuts off each story halfway . . . to be continued, for a thousand nights. A number of the stories mention hashish. In "The Tale of the Hashish Eater," a man eats hashish, goes to the public bath, falls asleep there, and has erotic fantasies that cause him to awaken with his hand on his erection amid the laughter of onlookers. In a second story, a hashish eater exiting the public bath passes an attractive young man entering, does an about-face, and follows him back in. (The green one made him do it.) In a third hashish-in-the-public-bath story (this one not from *One Thousand and One Nights*) the hashish-eating patron walks out of the bath wearing a towel, enters a second bath unaware of what he's doing, and, at the end of the afternoon, can't find his clothes. A crowd leads him naked through the street back to the first bath, shouting "hurrah for hashish."

Overall, the common denominator of such popular stories involving hashish eaters is foolishness. Hashish makes people lose touch with reality, and the result is silly and undignified. So, did you hear the one about the hashish eater who went out for grapes and barley? He gave the grapes to his donkey and the barley to his wife! There are several stories about hashish eaters mistaking the glow of moonlight for water on the ground. One tells of a poet who, having recited his poetry at a gathering of hashish eaters, goes out into the moonlit street. The moonlight shines on the ground, and thinking that it has inexplicably flooded, the poet hikes up his robe to keep it dry. Passersby witness his indignity and make fun of him. Another hashish eater, mistaking the moonlight for water, tries to dive into it. Hashish eaters? They could mistake a camel for a gnat!

The effects of hashish per se, it seems fair to say, did not seem very *threatening* to the disapproving majority. Medieval Arabic sources never suggest that hashish eating led to criminal behavior, much less violence (not even theft to pay for the drug), despite its being considered strongly habit-forming. The distaste directed at hashish seems to derive more from associated patterns of deviance, such as religious dissidence and homosexuality (whether real or imagined), and from prejudice against non–Arabic-speaking peoples who lived somewhat (*not* far enough!) to the east.

Arabic sources associated hashish especially with these non-Arabic speakers. According to our list of hashish synonyms, nicknames, and code words, Turks called the green one *esrar*, meaning "secrets," and they made frequent use of it. Persians called it *shadanaj*, which could be translated as "royal grain," or, perhaps, "queen of insanity," and they made frequent use of it, too. The Sunni legal treatises written to counteract the popularity of hashish in the 1200s and 1300s agree that hashish came to the Muslim world from the east. That meant, in the first place, from Persia, where hashish almost certainly predated Islam itself. One anti-hashish legal treatise grumbled: "It was an evil restricted to Persia until the Tatars took it over. Then it moved on to Baghdad." By "Tatars" the author meant people from Central Asia then entering the eastern Muslim world in repeated waves, most recently Turks and Mongols. The great door through which they entered Muslim lands was the space between the Himalayas and the Aral Sea, the region of modern Turkmenistan and Uzbekistan. Here the Muslim world met the fearsome nomadic horse archers of Central Asia.

Central Asian conquerors took control of most of the Muslim world between the 1100s and the 1500s, and horse archers were the key to their success. Eventually, Muslim armies developed their own elite corps of horse archers, called *mamluks*. Mamluks were mercenaries who were, or had been, slaves. Normally, mamluks began as adolescent boys born and raised on the Central Asian steppes beyond the borders of Islam, where they had learned to ride and to use a bow on horseback from early childhood. Captured or sold into slavery, they were taken to Iraq or Syria or Egypt and shaped into disciplined troops. Separated forever from their kin, mamluks became Muslims but were normally kept separate from the Arabic speakers around them, often speaking Turkish instead. Once fully trained, mamluks were normally manumitted but remained devoted to their masters. Thus, they were not only militarily potent but politically convenient—disciplined and professional, with no families, and, therefore, undivided loyalty to their commander, at least in theory.

The sway of these foreign mercenaries multiplied after 1000 as the Muslim world fragmented politically and invaders entered from east and west. Sometimes, as in Egypt, mamluks seized power and created their own dynasties. Then, in the mid-1200s there was another knock at the door beyond the Caspian Sea, announcing another visitor from the steppes of Central Asia. It was Genghis Khan. The Mongols were not Muslims, not in a hurry to convert, and they had created arguably the most effective army in history. Their capture of Bagdad in 1258 destroyed the caliphate forever. Eventually, though, like the Seljuk Turks before them and the Ottoman Turks after them, the Mongols *did* convert. By around 1500, dynasties of Central Asian origin ruled practically the entire Muslim world.

The people of Baghdad, Damascus, and Cairo saw mamluks become a routine fixture of military power, and they learned to accept new Central Asian overlords, but it was a painful process. When anti-hashish treatises in Arabic blast Turks and Mongols for bringing hashish, their accusation must be understood in this larger context. Almost certainly, the accusation was true. The cannabis plant had first evolved in Central Asia. Eventually, we will follow it back to its geographic roots. For now, however, let us turn to the religious dissidents, some of whom placed themselves squarely outside Sunni traditions. They are the lead players in our story.

GOD'S UNRULY FRIENDS

The men called *Sufis* accepted the Qur'an and thought of themselves as "God's Friends," but they were unruly friends. Mainstream Sunnis regarded Sufis with stern disapproval, and only partly because some Sufis ate hashish. In general, Sufis took a contrasting approach to religion, scorning the proprieties of Sunni Muslim society.

From the first, Islam contained both world-renouncing and world-embracing, both prophetic and legalist, currents. The Qur'an exhorted Muslims to look beyond mundane concerns and lift their eyes toward heaven, but it also provided detailed instructions on how to live a Godly life on earth. One could say that the Qur'an is largely devoted to providing those instructions. The creation of a divinely ordered society was perhaps the central impulse of Muhammad's prophecy. The result was a powerful social and religious emphasis on law. After the Qur'an, the primary basis for Islamic law were the words and deeds of Muhammad, called *sunna,* and these are not recorded in the Qur'an. Instead, they were derived from many sources, principally oral traditions that were painstakingly verified and eventually written down as hadiths. Commentary on the sunna was the primary occupation of religious scholars in what we now call Sunni society. The firmly world-embracing Sunni outlook was majority and mainstream in the medieval Muslim world.

And yet, there were always world-renouncers—people disposed to withdraw from society and seek a different spiritual path. These were the Sufis, whose name refers to the rough wool cloak they wore, scorning comfort. They are often described as "mystics," but what most helps to understand them is their radical rejection of the whole Sunni approach to religion, including, notably, its legalism. Sunnis tried to live Godly lives in society, and their accumulated legal writings supplied a complex web of guidelines for doing so. Sufis turned their backs on society and its laws. Sufis put their energies into a daily quest for a direct encounter with divinity, somewhat as did the Christian friars of medieval Europe. Like European friars, Sufis might withdraw into the wilderness, subsist on alms, and devote all their time to prayer and meditation. They might live together, forming a Sufi order that could multiply its houses and spread geographically over time. The founders of particular Sufi orders were spiritual teachers who prescribed a particular way of seeking to know God—such as meditative techniques—and attracted followers who adopted the same techniques. These Sufi masters were regarded as saints after death, and their tombs became centers of veneration and pilgrimage. Like the Prophet Muhammad, Sufi masters claimed no divinity for themselves; rather, they were men who helped other men find God. More than dissidents disposed to argue against the Sunni rules, Sufis were nonconformists who simply ignored the rules.

During the 800s and 900s, when the word *hashish* still referred merely to animal fodder or garden weeds, Sufism had become a familiar and tolerated part of the Muslim world. Gradually, new Sufi orders appeared, particularly in non–Arabic-speaking regions, such as Persia and Sindh, at the western margin of India. In the 1200s, a new religious practice grew out of Sufism and went beyond it. The new practitioners redoubled the world-renouncing tendencies present among Sufis, utterly denying themselves the comforts of a normal life and rejecting social norms in their spiritual quest. Because the redoubled ascetic practice arose among Sufis, the practitioners were still Sufis in the view of outsiders. Yet because they were reacting against the respectable Sufism of their day (partly by eating hashish), we need a different name for them: dervishes. You may have heard of the whirling variety of dervishes, and now you know what set them whirling.

The two most important dervish groups were called Haydaris and Qalandars. Like earlier Sufis, dervishes were followers of particular spiritual teachers whose teachings outlived them. The Haydaris were followers of the Persian master named Qutb al-Din Haydar. In the mid-1100s, Haydar renounced the world and withdrew from society to live in the wilderness. The legend of his "discovery" of hashish has often been repeated. One day, the story goes, Haydar noticed that a particular plant swayed as if in the breeze, and yet there was no breeze. Curious, he ate some of the plant, which was cannabis, of course, and he found the result enlightening. Thereafter, Haydar taught his followers to eat hashish, saying that it held spiritual "secrets." He directed his followers to plant hashish around his tomb, so that pilgrims who came to visit it would find a ready supply.

Haydar's single-handed "discovery" of hashish in 1155 is the stuff of legend. In truth, the people of northeastern Persia, at the doorstep of Central Asia, where Haydar supposedly discovered hashish, already knew all about it. In addition to Persians, many of his early followers were Turkic speakers who were entering Persia from Central Asia in these years. Haydar's followers multiplied and spread their practice west to Iraq, Syria, and Egypt. They were not the only dervishes, either.

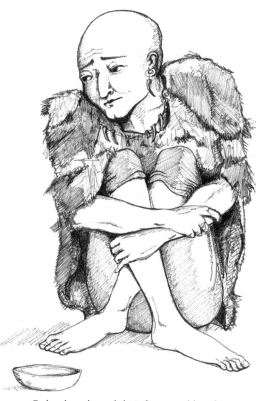

Qalandars shaved their faces and heads.

A second dervish order, the Qalandars, focused on a second Persian master, Jamal al-Din Savi, who preached in Damascus in the 1100s and who also appears, in the literature of later centuries, as a "discoverer" of hashish. This holy man's ascetic quest led him to reside in a cemetery, whereby he enacted his central teaching. Qalandars were to "die before their death," renouncing the world to become social nonentities. Jamal al-Din Savi went practically naked, which exposed him to the elements and (another benefit) kept people away. Still, he acquired followers in Syria and his teaching spread to Egypt.

The world upon which Haydaris and Qalandars turned their backs was a specifically Sunni world. Renouncing family and a normal social life, they also rejected the Sunni rules for living, the shari'a, with its comprehensive guidelines for everything from civil and criminal law to diet and personal hygiene. Dervishes flaunted their disregard for normal Muslim proprieties and adopted an intentionally outrageous appearance. Rather than wearing full beards as medieval Muslim men normally did, Qalandars did the opposite. They shaved their faces, their heads, even their eyebrows. Haydaris could be recognized by their iron collars, bracelets, and anklets that symbolized their spiritual self-discipline and mortification of the flesh. Usually not visible, thanks to minimal clothing (made of hides or leaves, for example) were the iron rings that Haydaris wore on their genitals as guarantees of chastity. Dervishes symbolized their rejection of human society by adorning themselves with bones, horns, and strings of animal teeth. They played drums and bells as they moved through the streets. While they traveled extensively, they seldom made the pilgrimage to Mecca that the Qur'an lists among the obligations of devout Muslims.

Having "died before their deaths," dervishes blithely disregarded the religious duties of the living. They conspicuously failed to fast during the month of Ramadan. They would happily drink wine, but wine was an expensive luxury, and dervishes were mendicants who carried a begging bowl. Hashish, on the other hand, they could afford. The "daughter of the bag" fit the wandering dervish life perfectly. It eased privations, gladdened the heart, and made one want to sing and dance. The Sunni legislative reaction against hashish clearly associated it with dervishes, and also with some formerly respectable Sufis who had taken up aspects of dervish practice as it spread through the Arabic-speaking center of the Muslim world. Arabic *ma'lum*, roughly "the poor Sufi's compensation," became one of the more widely recognized nicknames for hashish.

As the stories about Haydar suggest, the dervishes (and eventually other Sufis) used hashish not only to ease privations and gladden the heart but also in religious meditation. A Qalandar source gives precise, though plainly idealized, instructions for the ritual. The virtuous man who wishes to use this drug, which, being lawful, is better than wine, should purify himself beforehand, in spirit, body, and clothing. He should find an appropriate place, whether alone or in the company of others who share the secret. A place with murmuring water is best. He should hold the hashish in his right hand and ask for access to its insights in a lengthy speech that amounts, in summary paraphrase, to the following: "I am asking God, Who art generous with both rich and poor, all-powerful and omniscient, Who brought forth the grass of the field, created this secret, and disclosed it to those worthy of knowing it, to allow me its use, protecting me from harm, that I may see things as they really are." The Qalandar was then to chew and swallow the hashish, and rinse the remnants from his mouth before chanting the praise of the Creator. He was to whiten his teeth with antimony, removing tell-tale signs of the green one, so that the uninitiated would not discover his secret. As the effect took hold, he was to remain serene in demeanor and moderate in both speech and action, seeking the most delicate food, the most beautiful surroundings, and the most instructive company, meditating upon cause and effect, upon doer and deed, upon the speaker and the words spoken, seeking to understand the eternal knowledge of God and his universal grace, thus becoming a little more separate from humanity and moving a little closer to divinity. A Sufi poet wrote that the green one "made his house into a mosque."

Hashish fit the Sufi emphasis on ecstatic experience. Spiritual intoxication, music, and dance, because they diverted one from the ordinary world, enabled the mystical quest for nearness to God. Unlike most Muslims, Sufis incorporated music into their poetic liturgies, which they chanted in unison. Voice and words, rather than instruments or harmony, constituted the main elements of their music. Sufi music thus stemmed from recitation of the Qur'an and other standard Muslim prayers, such as the innumerable names of God. But music encouraged rapture, leading some participants to dance spontaneously for joy. Contemporary "whirling dervishes" do a controlled dance-meditation that grows out of this tradition.

Sufi poetry was occasionally dedicated to hashish. More often, however, it was dedicated to wine or to a lover, in the general tradition of Arabic and Persian poetry. Among Sufis, such poetry was interpreted metaphorically, rather as the Song of Solomon, apparently a love lyric, has been interpreted religiously by Jews and Christians as symbolizing love of God. One way or another, Sufism channeled some of the finest artistic impulses in the medieval Muslim world. The great poet Rumi was a Persian-born Sufi with Haydari and Qalandar associates. Followers of Rumi founded the Mevlevi order, the renowned "whirling dervishes" of today. Still, the themes of love and intoxication, chanted and danced in a Sufi lodge, raised straitlaced Sunni suspicions of drug-induced mysticism, which they considered not one bit Muslim.

Sunni jurists were angered by the religious use of hashish. They expressed concern about secret use in mosques and refuted the claim (of a Sufi poet) that its usefulness is greater than the sin of using it. Ibn Tammiyyah, author of one of the principal anti-hashish treatises, believed that hashish had entered the Arabic-speaking world with the Mongols, and he compared the religious use of hashish to certain practices of Christians, practices which, in his view, however much the Christians might believe in them, were simply not the correct way to worship God. And if the Sunni religious establishment did not know the correct way to worship God, it knew nothing at all. It thoroughly mistrusted ecstatic inspiration and charismatic masters. The accumulated, collective wisdom of its religious jurists was the heart of Sunni authority.

Questioning authority, on the other hand, was what the more radical Sufis were all about. The Abdals, a later dervish order in what is now Turkey, were apparently full of young runaways who had broken ties with their elders. The student who had quarreled with his teacher, the beardless youth defying his father—these were the sorts who might be seduced away to join the Abdals. Outlandishly dressed, singing and dancing to mystical music, jeering at military commanders and judges, the young Abdals proclaimed that "they would not be true to the Truth" if they failed to annoy "the people of the Law." They seem to have succeeded very well at exasperating their elders and the authorities in general.

In the period 1100–1500, then, mainstream Muslim society was beleaguered by numerous challengers (religious nonconformists from within, invaders from without) whom it associated with hashish. Sufis and dervishes, with their outrageous attire, or lack of it, may appear innocuous from a modern viewpoint, but from the medieval Sunni perspective they were seriously heretical. Consider also that the associations with "recreational" hashish eating—including poverty, sexual deviance, and a general lack of respectability—were far from glamorous. It will then be unsurprising that "hashish eater" became a common slur.

With that slur in mind, and with an understanding of various tensions around hashish in medieval Muslim society, let us return to the mentioned 1123 document in which the word *hashish*—actually, the word *hashish eater*—first enters the historical record. The targets of the slur in the 1123 document were the most famous hashish eaters ever, the legendary Assassins.

THE ASSASSIN LEGEND

Harry Anslinger featured a popular version of the Assassin legend in his 1930s campaign to make marijuana illegal throughout the United States. To clarify the connection between marijuana, madness, and murder, Anslinger explained that the very word *assassin* came from *hashish*, and he told a chilling tale of an elite corps of medieval Muslim assassins who consumed hashish to launch their bloody attacks. Most of his story came from his own imagination, and other people's, because this legend had been embroidered over many centuries. The word *assassin* in English and many other European languages does indeed derive from the Arabic word *hashishiyya*, hashish eaters. Many other aspects of the Assassin legend have little basis in reality. But can it be that, as many believe today, history's most famous hashish eaters never really ate hashish at all?

Let's begin with the legend itself, which circulated widely in Europe thanks to *The Travels of Marco Polo*. On his way to China in the mid-1200s, the celebrated Venetian traveler had passed through Syria and Persia, where he heard about a sect that specialized in assassinating enemy leadership. In an age when poison was the preferred agent of political murder, these specialist "ashishin" (as Polo rendered their name) killed only with a dagger, first gaining the confidence of the enemy leader, infiltrating his entourage, wait-ing patiently for an opportunity to get close, and finally striking before the victim's bodyguards could react. The assassins rarely escaped after killing their victims, though. What astounded their enemies was their discipline and devotion, as one can sense from another "ashishin" story, wherein a sentry on a high castle rampart unhesitatingly hurls himself into the abyss when commanded to do so. Many such stories circulated, apparently. The one related by Marco Polo attributed the group's spectacular devotion to its Syr-ian leader, the Old Man of the Mountain, who reputedly recruited young men to be assassins by giving them a mysterious drink that made them lose consciousness. The young men awakened in a delightful garden where they envisioned the reward that awaited martyrs in heaven.

Marco Polo's account of the group was not the first to reach Western Europe. Writing in the early 1200s, a German chronicler of the Third Crusade had already described the Old Man of the Mountain's use of a vision-producing potion that showed recruits the delights that would be eternally theirs if they died for the cause. Many accounts of the group make no mention of a potion, but they still call them "hashish eaters." During the high point of the group's activities in the 1100s, it seems, that was how the group was generally known, to Christians and Muslims alike.

The reality behind the Assassin legend, as applied by Anslinger and others, may go no further than that. The slur *hashish eater* may have been directed at the followers of the Old Man of the Mountain in exactly the spirit that the English slur *bastard* might be hurled without any real thought to anyone's paternity. But maybe there's more to it.

Remember, this was an *Arabic* slur, directed at Muslims by other Muslims. The objects of the slur, the real people behind the As-sassin legend, have a considerable and well-documented history. They do not lack a real name. The Nizari Ismailis were religious dissenters, as were the Sufis, but whereas Sufis merely thumbed their noses at the Sunni establishment, Nizari Ismailis wanted to overthrow it. From a Sunni perspective, they were much more menacing.

Nizari dissidence sprang from an ongoing dispute about who represented the legitimate succession of the Prophet Muhammad in the centuries after his death, which means that Nizaris belonged to the Shi'a branch of Islam. Muhammad was a political and military, in addition to a spiritual, leader. For roughly five hundred years after Muhammad, leaders called *caliphs* represented his authority over the entire Muslim world, but only in theory. In fact, the explosive growth of Islam quickly outran the ability of any caliph to rule over it from Baghdad, which was the principal seat of the caliphate. Only the first few caliphs were universally recognized. Descent from the Prophet's family offered the strongest claim to the caliphate, but Muhammad had left no male heir and, inevitably, conflicting claims appeared.

Without entering into a detailed discussion of particular claims—who successively became caliph, violating the more legitimate claim of whomever—let us observe the conflict so to comprehend the true identity of the Nizaris and, above all, the radical and subversive nature of their anti-Sunni dissidence. The nature of their dissidence bears directly, as you will see, on the matter of whether the Nizaris actually ate hashish.

When an "illegitimate" candidate became caliph, the result, in the eyes of dissenters, was a religious catastrophe. The throne of God's representative on earth had been usurped, and things would be out of kilter until the rightful heir of the Prophet recovered the throne. In the meantime, each new caliph of the illegitimate line would be a usurper, too, and the gradual construction of religious law built up during the reign of usurper caliphs, as well as all their appointments and decisions, would lack legitimacy. Therefore, the apparently limited and specific disagreement about who should have become caliph centuries ago effectively alienated dissenting Shi'a Muslims from the dominant religious and political power structure of Sunni Islam. Shiites became a sort of permanent opposition party. And since their belief found less expression in the law (which belonged mostly to the Sunni power structure), it focused instead on the authority of charismatic leaders who often claimed descent from the Prophet. In fact, Shi'a Muslims espoused an alternative lineage of caliphs-in-waiting, whom they called the *imams*. The Shi'a main branch counted twelve known imams and awaited news of the next still-unknown one, termed "the hidden imam." The faithful believed that the hidden imam would appear one day to reclaim the caliphate, which more or less never happened. Instead, Shiites remained a powerless and frustrated minority almost everywhere in the Muslim world, the greatest exception being Persia.

The Persian Nizaris were a splinter group that represented a split (actually two successive splits) within Shi'a ranks. Nizaris accepted only the first seven of the "twelve known imams." After that, they recognized a different lineage of imams starting with one named Ismail, hence Nizari *Ismailis*. People dissatisfied with the existing order tended to gravitate toward Shi'a groups, and especially toward the Ismailis, because of their looking-for-a-change orientation. Ismaili beliefs were notably changeable, often unorthodox, and above all, secret, revealed only to initiates. Ismailis admitted a metaphorical reading of the Qur'an, and, like Sufis, they had a tendency to disregard the accumulated tradition of Sunni religious law-giving. Compared with other Shiites, Ismailis challenged the mainstream Sunni order more aggressively. After gaining converts in Iraq, Persia, Yemen, and Syria, a Hidden Imam revealed himself and was able to establish an Ismaili caliphate in Egypt in the year 973. This was called the Fatimid dynasty because its legitimacy depended partly on claims of descent from the Prophet's daughter, Fatima. The Fatimid caliphate dominated Egypt for two centuries, a major eruption of Shi'a power in the heartland of Sunni Islam. The Nizaris broke away from other Ismailis when their candidate for Fatimid caliph was murdered in 1095.

Now that we have a better view of the Nizaris, we can better understand the motivations of both the Nizari assassins and their detractors. Although they did assassinate one high-profile Christian crusader prince, the Nizaris' main targets were other Muslims, the Seljuk Turks who were just then taking over the Baghdad caliphate and the Sunni power structure that went with it. The Sunnis regarded the Nizari assassinations as treacherous and ignoble, so they might well hurl an insult into the teeth of the Nizaris: "Hashishiyya! Riffraff! Lowly hashish eaters!" Rare is the blood enemy not tagged with an insulting name, after all.

But why this particular name? Shi'a groups did have a reputation for attracting poor and marginal people, so that may account for the "lowly" part. But Arabic is not without meaningful insults to hurl at an enemy. Why call the Nizaris *hashish eaters* if the term lacked specificity in their case? And if it was a random insult, in which the particular content of the slur was irrelevant, then why did it stick so powerfully? After all, we are not trying to understand how an angry person could call the Nizaris "hashish eaters" in a moment of pique. To the contrary, this derisive nickname for the group became so widely known that many European witnesses (not catching the reference to hashish) thought it was a proper name.

That suggests more than a random insult.

Let's reason carefully here. No historical source gives any indication that Nizari assassins consumed *any* drug to carry out their assassinations. The Nizari assassin was a one-man sleeper cell, whose entire efficacy depended on escaping the slightest suspicion as he gained the confidence of his target. In all credible sources that specifically mention a drug (and many do not), the drug merely attracts new recruits with visions of a heavenly reward. Its main effect is to put them to sleep. No source names hashish, except of course, by insistently calling the Nizaris "hashish eaters."

On the other hand, Arabic speakers had every reason to view the Nizaris as Persians, and they associated hashish with Persia, as we have seen. The Nizari leadership was unquestionably Persian, and their liturgical language seems to have been Persian, too, rather than Arabic. Although the Nizaris had a Syrian offshoot (the most famous for its daring assassinations), they were in fact primarily a Persian group. Furthermore, the group's stronghold lay in *northeast* Persia (on the doorstep of Central Asia), the same area where Haydar supposedly "discovered" hashish and founded the dervish order that made his name synonymous with hashish.

Also very salient for Arabic speakers was the group's radical religious dissidence. In their commitment to worldly struggle, not to mention their violent tactics, the Nizaris were totally unlike the contemplative Sufis. Still, both were *antinomians* (*nomos* is Greek for *law*), which means that neither had much time for Sunni proprieties and prohibitions. For the Nizaris, the reappearance of the Hidden Imam could trigger a totally new dispensation, under which the faithful would no longer be bound by the old religious laws at all. For example, in the year 1164, the group's Persian leader, ensconced in one of the Nizaris' impregnable castles built on mountain peaks, proclaimed a message from the Hidden Imam, whose revelation he indicated to be imminent. According to Nizari accounts, to make the proclamation the leader assembled the faithful as if to pray—but facing away from Mecca, instead of toward it. He then invited them to feast during what had been, until that moment, a time of obligatory fasting. The Nizaris' new legal dispensation was announced in Syria that same year, and hostile Sunni sources there reported scandalous debauchery, incest, and wine drinking after the announcement. They did not mention hashish. Perhaps they did not have to.

In sum, it seems inescapable that, whether by ethnic profiling or because of religious prejudice, the Arabic-speaking Sunni enemies of the Nizaris *did* associate them with hashish, and not merely as a random slur. Surely that is why the Arabic nickname "hashish eaters" stuck to them so firmly. Given what we've learned about the historical context, the idea was hardly absurd, whether prejudiced or not. Yet hashish was a symptom, not a cause of the Sunni quarrel with the Nizaris. The Sunni legal establishment had not yet passed collective judgment on hashish as a drug in the 1100s. When that happened gradually in the 1200s and 1300s, the Nizari assassins were irrelevant to the discussion. The notion that hashish could directly incite violence seems quite absent from the medieval Muslim world.

NOT FOR EVERYBODY

The Muslim world's experience with psychotropic cannabis, spanning centuries and continents, is a key piece of the drug's global history. The main lesson I glean from it is that, historically, cannabis drugs have never been for everybody.

As in the Atlantic World, cannabis users in the Muslim world tended to be marginal in some way. They were often religious or philosophical nonconformists and poor laborers, often ethnically distinct from the majority. As in the United States, the most famous cannabis users of the Muslim world were flamboyant cultural dissidents who marginalized themselves from mainstream society and who believed that the drug helped them gain spiritual insights. There is something undeniably hippielike about the early dervishes, with their outrageous appearance, their peripatetic lifestyle, their declarations of universal peace and love, and their gleeful going against the grain of mainstream society, disregarding its conventions and taboos, refusing to recognize the legitimacy of its constituted authorities.

Clearly, the prohibition of alcohol for observant Muslims did *not* create societies that ate hashish the way Europeans drank wine and beer. According to UN figures, annual prevalence of cannabis use in the Muslim world is 1 to 3 percent today. While generally disapproving, Muslim attitudes toward hashish have been mostly tolerant, however. Over centuries, eating (and later, smoking) hashish got users in trouble, but not *too much* trouble. Despite the stark rhetoric of anti-hashish jurists, the green one was tolerated as a minor vice, less sinful than wine, less apt to result in violence, and always, less expensive than alcohol, which remained the euphoriant of choice, insofar as we can tell. Once established in the years 1100–1500, that general pattern apparently lasted more or less until the twentieth century, when international agreements resulted in a more restrictive climate.

The sprawling community of Muslim faithful converged at the crossroads of Europe, Asia, and Africa, the world's grand historical bazaar of cultural innovations, when hashish appeared in it around 1100. It was from there that psychoactive cannabis spread around the world. When "modern hashish" (the concentrated resin of many plants) appeared more recently, it too spread through the Muslim world and became largely identified with it. The hashish that went to Europe and even, eventually, the United States seems to have carried with it the dreamy, tolerant ethos of Egyptian Sufism.

French soldiers noticed hashish in Egypt when Napoleon took an army there, disastrously, in 1798, and they returned with it to

France, where it briefly became part of a vogue for things exotic and "Oriental." Europeans wanted Chinese silks and porcelains, Persian carpets, and a nice cup of that exotic drink, tea. They wanted to read *One Thousand and One Nights* in sensational translations, and also the provocative verses of Omar Khayyam, a Persian mathematician and astronomer whose successful free translation into English made his poetry better known in that language than in Persian. Just as alcohol represented Europe in this way of thinking, opium represented China, and hashish represented the Muslim world. Europe's most avant-garde writers wondered what they could learn from both opium and hashish.

Hashish eating in the 1800s was confined to a few bohemians and free-thinking artists and writers, especially French and English, in search of exotic experience and stimulus to the imagination. The roll call of participants is short but impressive. Honoré de Balzac and Victor Hugo, two of the most important French writers of the century, belonged to a Parisian Hashish Eaters' Club in the 1840s. Club members, who sometimes wore turbans to enhance the mood, reported *synesthesia*—seeing sounds, hearing colors—and described magic-carpet voyages and spectacular visions that were presumably worth all the effort: "My eyelashes grew ever longer without stopping and, like gold thread, rolled up on small ivory spinning wheels." Others who certainly experimented with hashish included Charles Baudelaire and Arthur Rimbaud. So, probably, did Alexandre Dumas, who has a hugely exoticizing description of a hashish experience in *The Count of Monte Cristo*. Altering consciousness was a Romantic predilection, one might say.

Hashish had a parallel but more limited nineteenth-century vogue in the United States, where there were fewer young aristocrats to destroy themselves with tragic abandon. A 1850s *Atlantic Monthly* travelogue recounted the experience of eating hashish in Damascus, and a young man from Poughkeepsie, New York, experimented with double doses of Tilden's Extract, a patent medicine containing hashish, then described his terrifying visions in a book, *The Hasheesh Eater*. Even a Louisa May Alcott story, "Perilous Play," warned fashionable girls away from hashish confections in 1869. There was a Turkish Hashish Pavilion at Philadelphia's

Centennial Exposition in 1876. *Harper's Magazine* even reported on a Hashish Parlor, something like an upscale opium den, where "male and female patrons of the better class" sampled hashish confections in 1883 New York. Hashish extracts like Tilden's were easily available in U.S. pharmacies, but how widely isn't clear. Certainly, they were not as popular as extracts from opium. Although various opium extracts became quite standard nineteenth-century pain killers (also used as soporifics and antidiarrhetics), most people in the United States had still barely heard of hashish around 1900 when marijuana cigarettes appeared in the brown hands of migrant farm workers and New Orleans stevedores. Even people who had heard of both hashish and marijuana found it difficult to make the connection between dreamy hashish and "the killer weed."

Whether in a hashish confection or a marijuana cigarette, though, cannabis drugs weren't for everyone in the twentieth-century United States, or anywhere else in the Atlantic World. They have never been exactly "normal," anywhere, it seems, even when not illegal. Hashish was certainly never "normal" in the medieval Muslim world. The poor who resorted to the green one instead of wine couldn't afford to be "normal," so to speak, and Sufis, who regarded hashish as mind-expanding, had no wish to be.

But what about India? If cannabis drugs were normal in any society throughout their history, surely it was India. Promoters of marijuana have confidently claimed that it was "the wine of India." And how about Central Asia, the place where cannabis originates and where human beings first used it?

5

✳

Asian Origins

This chapter traces the origins of cannabis back to prehistoric Central Asia. Our most intense scrutiny will go to the Indian subcontinent, where cannabis drugs have a three-thousand-year history. Then we will see how the cannabis plant was transported around prehistoric Central Asia by steppe nomads who applied it to their funeral rites. Finally, we'll consider what people were apparently doing with psychoactive cannabis before the dawn of civilization.

HISTORIC INDIA

India is the proverbial home of cannabis drugs, which is why the U.S. counterculture sought inspiration there. Allen Ginsberg's 1966 *Atlantic Monthly* manifesto, "The Great Marijuana Hoax," aptly exemplifies the counterculture's general view of India. Ginsberg wrote this passage while smoking marijuana to illustrate its effects:

In sound good health I smoked legal ganja (as marijuana is termed in India, where it is traditionally used in preference to alcohol), bought from government tax shops in Calcutta, in a circle of devotees, yogis, and hymn-singing pious Shaivite worshipers in the burning ground at Nimtallah Ghat in Calcutta, where it was the custom of these

respected gentlemen to meet on Tues. and Saturday nights, smoke
before an improvised altar of blossoms, sacramental milk-candy &
perhaps a fire taken from the burning wooden bed on which lay
a newly dead body, of some friend perhaps, likely a stranger if a
corpse is a stranger, pass out the candy as God's gift to friend and
stranger, and sing holy songs all night, with great strength and
emotion, addressed to different images of the Divine Spirit. Ganja
was there considered a beginning of sadhana (Yogic path or discipline) by some; others consider the Ascetic Yogi Shiva Himself to
have smoked marijuana; on His birthday marijuana is mixed as a
paste with almond milk by the grandmothers of pious families and
imbibed as a sacrament by this polytheistic nation, considered by
some a holy society. The professors of English at Benares University
brought me a bottle for the traditional night of Shivaratri, birthday
of the Creator & Destroyer who is the patron god of this oldest con-
tinuously inhabited city on Earth. "BOM BOM MAHADEV!" (Boom
Boom Great God!) is the Mantra Yogis cry as they raise the ganja
pipe to their brows before inhaling.

Ginsberg has real knowledge of his topic, obviously, and he's quite
correct in linking ganja, the great Hindu deity Shiva, and the holy
men he calls *yogis*—but his description greatly exaggerates the role
of cannabis drugs in Indian civilization. Popular histories of marijuana have perpetuated this error for half a century. In fact, good
information on cannabis drugs in India is amazingly scarce before
the twentieth century.

India's cannabis drugs came to the attention of modern Europeans early in the age of European seaborne imperialism and colonization, when sailors and explorers sent back reports of a cannabis
drink called *bhang*, a word that the reader may recall. An early
Portuguese chronicler in India, Garcia da Orta, remarked that his
Indian servants told him bhang improved their mood, stimulated
their appetite, and helped them work. "I believe that it is so generally used and by such a number of people that there is no mystery
about it," he wrote. During the period of British colonial rule in
India, cannabis drugs were regulated and taxed. In fact, a British
colonial study, the 1893–1894 *Report of the Indian Hemp Drugs Commission*, is often cited as the most serious large-scale social study

of marijuana ever undertaken. The commission found that "hemp drugs" did not constitute a social problem and should not be outlawed. Still, as with hashish in the Muslim world, the prevalence of cannabis drugs in India has been blown out of proportion by the Western imagination.

Indians of the 1890s distinguished systematically between various cannabis drugs and held contrasting opinions about them. For starters, there was *ganja*, a Hindi word we have already encountered in Jamaica; ganja was the flowering top of the female plant. Next, there was *charas*; charas was the concentrated resin of many flowering tops, what is today called "hashish." But the most important cannabis drug in Indian history is undoubtedly *bhang*, the drink described by Garcia da Orta. To make the bhang drink, Indians traditionally used the leaves of the entire plant, washed, boiled, and ground to a pulp. They added a spice mix including saffron, rose petals, poppy seeds, black pepper, dried ginger, caraway, clove, cinnamon, cucumber seeds, melon seeds, cardamom, almonds, pistachio, or nutmeg, and finally sugar. Both the bhang pulp and spice paste were then combined with liquid. The liquid necessarily included milk, rich with butter fat, that gradually became infused with cannabinoids as the bhang simmered for many hours before being strained and chilled. Ice cream can be made with similar ingredients, as can various green psychoactive confections, which Ginsberg described on Shiva's birthday.

Bhang is also the Indian name of the whole cannabis plant, a name transplanted with that meaning to the Swahili coast of Africa. One of the most ancient Indian sacred texts, the Atharva Veda, mentions the bhang plant. The Atharva Veda was composed before 1000 BCE. That's one thousand years before the Common Era, which is to say over three thousand years ago, a meaningful duration even on the scale of global history. By grouping bhang with the sacred hallucinogen *soma*, the Atharva Veda indicates its psychoactive powers. Vedic mention of cannabis has often been used to signal the plant's deep roots in Indian life, and rightly so, at least regarding the antiquity of its ceremonial use. And yet, the next prominent mention of psychoactive cannabis in India comes a long, long time—twenty centuries—after the Atharva Veda.

Here's all the documentary evidence in a nutshell. From around 1000 BCE on, cannabis appears in a mere handful of existing written texts, mostly pharmacopeias, until the year 1050 CE, two thousand years later, when we get a list of Sanskrit synonyms for *bhang*. Then around the year 1300 we get another dribble of clues, nicknames suggestive of psychoactive use, including, in its earliest recorded appearance, the word *ganja*. In the 1500s, we get a few European reports, already mentioned. The main one is Garcia da Orta's description of the bhang drink:

> The profit from its use is for the man to be outside himself, and to be raised above all cares and anxieties, and it makes some break into a foolish laugh. I hear that many women take it when they want to dally and flirt with men. It is also said, but it may not be true, that the great captains, in ancient times, used to drink it with wine or with opium, that they might rest from their work, be without care, and be able to sleep; for the long vigils of such became a torment to them. The great Sultan Bahadur said to Martim Affonso de Souza, to whom he wished every good thing and to whom he told his secrets, that when at night he wanted to go to Portugal, Brazil, Turkey, Arabia, or Persia, he only had to take a little BANGUE.

And that's about all the primary-source evidence currently available in the world's libraries concerning the use of cannabis drugs in India before the 1800s. Much more could potentially be added by primary research in Indian languages, no doubt. For now, however, we have breathtakingly little evidence to represent centuries of a supposedly common practice.

What's going on? Indian kingdoms with elaborate, highly refined cultures and writing stretch back as far as civilization itself. References to wine are commonplace in early Hebrew, Greek, and Latin writing. What happened to the historical evidence of cannabis drugs in India? Part of the answer is that India's historical record as a whole is a bit sketchy when compared to other places. Indians have been reading and writing longer than any Europeans, but the earliest script has not yet been deciphered, and much of what historical Indians wrote has disappeared. The chief writing surface in classical India was, in fact, dried palm leaves. India's hot and humid climate eventually dissolved all palm leaf documents, along with the subcontinent's ancient wooden cities. Both written and physical traces of the past are consequently less abundant in India than in the Middle East, Europe, or China. Nonetheless, there are sources enough to say with confidence that, during the years when Hebrews, Greeks, and Romans were drinking all that wine, Indians were drinking wine, too.

Fermented drinks were very much on the scene in ancient India. The fabulous diversity of India—its thousands of deities and devotions, its society so compartmentalized by caste and region—allows only a few basic generalizations on this matter. Here they are. First, *bhang* definitely did *not* substitute for wine, which was plentiful in the cities of classical India. Modern India's dominant religions, both Hindu and Muslim, discourage alcohol consumption, but the dominant religion of classical India, roughly 500 BCE to 500 CE, was Buddhism, which concentrated its discipline on monasteries and, at least in practice, did not limit wine consumption among the general urban populace. Classical sources depict wine-drenched festivals, scenes of drunken revelry involving nobles, urban elites, prostitutes, entire communities. Dutiful housewives were instructed by the Kama Sutra to keep a bit of the good stuff (*wine*, mind you) on hand. Imported wine was uniformly the drink of royal courts, and India, normally divided into myriad small kingdoms, had many royal courts and droves of tipsy courtiers. Taverns flew banners to announce themselves. Classical Indian medical treatises praised wine at length. Classical Indians did not identify with wine the way that classical Greeks did, nor mass-produce it with Roman organizational zeal, but drink it with gusto they surely did. Buddhism declined and eventually disappeared from India about a thousand years ago. Thereafter, Indians (especially high-caste Brahmins) took an increasingly dim view of alcohol. Still, alcohol hardly vanished from Indian life, and the British promoted new forms of it.

Let us return, however, to our one rich and accessible pre-twentieth-century Indian source in English, the famous *Indian Hemp Drugs Commission Report* of the 1890s. The unique virtue of this source is that the commission tried systematically to find how and where cannabis grew in India, how it was regarded, how and where it was consumed, and by whom. Its information-gathering drew on thousands of witnesses over a period of years, and though the result is patchy, the broad outlines are clear. To begin, the commission found an enormous contrast between bhang (the drink) and ganja.

The bhang drink was consumed seasonally and communally. It was made mostly from cannabis that grew wild or with minimal cultivation. Because of this, and because it was usually made from the leaves of both male and female plants, the bhang drink was only mildly psychoactive. Customs varied regionally, as do all things Indian, and generally bhang was more northern than southern. The drink was a traditional accompaniment of celebrations, such as weddings. Certain religious festivals called for it specifically. On the last day of the Bengali festival of Durga Puja, for example, families offered cups of bhang to their guests, and all were expected "to partake thereof, or at least place it to the lips in token of acceptance," according to the 1890s commission report. Depending on the locality, just about everybody, up and down the social hierarchy, might drink bhang during a festival, and then might not drink it again for a year. It appears that men drank bhang more than did women, but bhang was often made and drunk in a domestic setting. Few considered it to be harmful.

Traditional patterns suggest that bhang-drinking may well have occurred in Indian villages from time immemorial. Bhang is made by the same basic technique—pounding, steeping, and straining—as prescribed by the Rig Veda for soma, the hallucinogenic drink of the priestly caste of preclassical India, more than three thousand years ago. Strainers that might have been used for the bhang drink have been found, too, by archeologists excavating Harappa and Mohenjo Daro, principal cities of the Indus Valley civilization (of modern Pakistan), unquestionably the earliest in South Asia, thriving a full millennium before the Rig Veda. Overall, the Indian Hemp Drugs Commission found the bhang drink integrated with many ancient and pervasive rhythms of Indian life. Most of the commission's informants believed outlawing bhang would be viewed, by Indians at large, as an unwarranted colonial repression of established tradition.

Ganja and charas, on the other hand, were something else again. Here, not to put too fine a point on it, were the serious drug users: men (exclusively) who tended to consume daily, usually by smoking ganja or charas in a stemless *chillum*. The chillum may have been invented by pulling the bowl off a hookah. Its unusual stemless shape requires a seemingly clumsy maneuver to smoke it while keeping it upright. But the maneuver gave the chillum an advantage in India. Smokers often passed a chillum around, and each smoker inhaled through his own cupped hand, not placing his lips on the pipe itself and thus avoiding an indirect contact forbidden by caste strictures.

The British had a particularly good grasp of who, and how many, smoked ganja because they licensed its production, supervised its distribution, and taxed its sale. (Clearly, this information is relevant to the commission's final decision not to prohibit cannabis drugs.) Their production took place entirely on "a compact tract having a radius of about sixteen miles," called the Ganja Mahal (I am not making that up), in what was then Bengal, today Bangladesh. There the ground was prepared meticulously, the plants trimmed to encourage growth of the flowering tops, and the males culled to prevent the females from going to seed. (Note that the Ganja Mahal produced *sin semilla*.) Bengal ganja was considered the best ganja in India, and the Ganja Mahal was the largest producer, sending its product across the entire north. Therefore, the commission was able to make quite informed estimates about the size of the consuming market, district by district, especially for the populous province of Bengal. By their calculation, the ganja-smoking population of rural districts was almost always under 1 percent, contrasting with urban Calcutta, at 5.4 percent. For the province as a whole, they estimated that ganja smokers amounted to something like one in fifty adult males.

One in fifty may be an undercount, of course. Still, the number is remarkably small by any standard. Unlike the "almost everybody" descriptions of occasional bhang drinking, ganja had a narrow social profile, according to the commission. Most generally, ganja users were men of the lower classes, whether Hindu or Muslim. They were village farmers, tradesmen, and artisans, fishermen and boatmen, day laborers and night watchmen. They were domestic servants of all kinds, such as laundrymen, doormen, porters, and the men who carried their "betters" through the dusty streets in covered sedan chairs. The report said that regular ganja use by such men was normally moderate and associated with their labors, and that, although clearly a marker of low social status, it was not considered a sign of particular dissipation. Aboriginal tribesmen and hill people all over India smoked ganja, too. And so, finally, did the wandering mendicants whom Ginsberg called *yogis*, men who made religious use of ganja.

The commission put these holy men first on its list of ganja smokers. We will call them *Sannyasins*, because the term expresses their world view. Sannyasins practice *sannyasa*, a basic concept of Hinduism. *Sannyasa* means the renunciation of a normal life, giving away one's possessions, withdrawing from society, and devoting oneself to prayer and spiritual discipline. Sannyasins try to disappear into the universe, become one with the cosmos, so to speak, even before death. Sound familiar? World renouncers, again, I'm afraid. In fact, the *fakirs* often mentioned in the *Commission Report* were basically Sufis in an Indian incarnation, Sufism being strongly present among the Muslims of the subcontinent. Indian Sannyasins shared a basic ascetic practice with historical Qalandars or Franciscan friars. All intentionally "mortified the flesh," seeking spiritual transcendence.

The ascetic practice of India was the oldest and biggest of all. Early Indian ascetics sometimes composed a substantial portion of the population. Buddhism (and possibly all later ascetic practices) emerged from this tradition. Among Hindus, world renouncers had links to the larger society because of the shared ideal of sannyasa. Sannyasa was the last stage of an ideal Hindu life, although ideal lives were surely no more common in ancient India than anywhere else. Still, all men except those of the lowest caste were supposed to become wandering mendicants at the end of their lives. Today, in popular parlance, India's wandering holy men are called *babas* (fathers, grandfathers). In the cultural scheme of ancient India, then, asceticism was a consensual religious value. Even those who didn't attempt it—most men didn't, women didn't at all—respected those

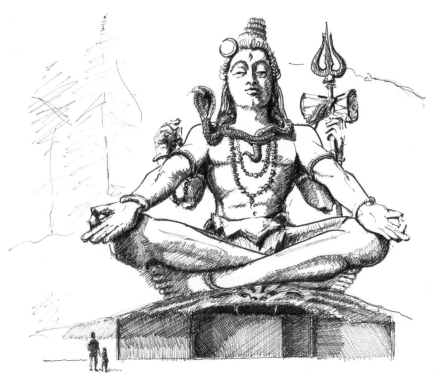

Shiva depicted as a meditating ascetic.

who did. In the 1890s, the commission reported that, in general, Indians were quite tolerant of the "grandfathers" who rarely bothered to conceal themselves from passersby when they huddled in a circle to share a chillum.

Babas sharing a chillum were likely to dedicate it to the awesome Lord Shiva, one of the three chief Hindu deities. An *alakh*, a ritual invocation pronounced with the first puff of a chillum, is today normally addressed to Shiva. It can be long or short, a summons, a request, a declaration of well-being, calling Shiva "Mahdeva," or Great Lord, and thereby acknowledging a special devotion. An anthropologist of the 1960s heard a baba say: "Hello Shiva, you come here. I want to one chillum together smoking." Importantly, Shiva was himself a practitioner of the ascetic arts, himself a yogi often depicted meditating in the lotus position. Ganja helped the

Sannyasins detach themselves from the world, meditate, and endure the physical privation of their sannyasa. Many nonascetic Indians also worship Shiva and drink bhang in his name. Shiva's luxuriant mythology has been embellished with stories declaring him Lord of Bhang and describing how he brought the plant down from the sacred mountain for the benefit of mankind.

The 1890s commission presented little information on charas, the most concentrated, and rarest, cannabis drug. Charas was used interchangeably with ganja in Punjab, the far northwest of the country. Elsewhere in India, however, it was virtually unknown. In fact, practically all charas seemed to be imported from outside India. Many of the commission's informants regarded charas as a new and not-very-Indian phenomenon. Unlike what we can see of bhang in the 1890s reportage, neither ganja nor charas conjures visions of Vedic continuities.

When did people learn to cull the male plants, trimming the females to stimulate the growth of their resinous buds, spacing them widely apart in full sun, and, no doubt, selectively breeding the most psychoactive strains, to make ganja? The word *ganja* appears in the historical record around 1300 CE, as already noted. That means sin semilla technique was invented more than a thousand years ago, but where and when? We'll have to look in Central Asia, because little more can be said, for now, about the history of cannabis drugs in India.

First, let's take stock of our Indian findings. We've identified a tradition of "normal," community-wide cannabis use, one spanning possibly three thousand years, in the traditional bhang drink of northern India. Historical bhang drinking was connected to religious observance, as during Durga Puja, but it was more for pleasure than insight, and thus basically recreational. Moreover, the Indian case has reaffirmed the historical affinity between cannabis drugs and poor laborers who use it to make simple, repetitive tasks more bearable. On the other hand, an ample majority of Indians, past and present, seem more likely to sample wine than any cannabis drug. Finally, we've found that the most dedicated users of ganja in historic India have been religious visionaries who intentionally sought the margin of normal life.

Indian myths say that Shiva brought the bhang plant down from the Himalayas that define the northern edge of the subcontinent. That makes sense, because the people whose sacred liturgies became the Vedas entered India themselves from the north around 1500 BCE. They were coming from the Eurasian steppes, a region that plays a surprisingly important role in our story.

THE PREHISTORIC EURASIAN STEPPES

Across Eurasia, from the Black Sea to Mongolia, stretch eight million square kilometers of plains too arid to support agriculture. From the perspective of the Atlantic World, the Eurasian steppes seem remote indeed—but they are actually central to global history. Psychoactive use of cannabis on and around the steppes is the oldest about which we have direct evidence. Among written sources, only Herodotus, the Greek "Father of History," has much to say about our topic, which is otherwise mostly prehistoric. Therefore, the following discussion will depend especially on archaeology. First, though, fascinating linguistic evidence helps get a fix on the Vedic people, who certainly brought psychoactive cannabis to India if it wasn't there already. To approach that evidence, we'll return momentarily to India, where a British scholar William Jones noticed something about Sanskrit as he studied the Vedas in the 1780s.

Jones believed that Sanskrit bore a clear family resemblance to Latin and Greek. He was quite correct. In fact, Sanskrit, along with the language of neighboring Iran, Farsi, bears a family resemblance to European languages in general. How did the resemblance come about? Scholars have been pondering that question for two centuries now. One of their tools has been "historical linguistics," a field of study that was invented, more or less, to address this very question. A family resemblance, the thinking goes, can only result from common descent. All the tongues in what historical linguists began to call—in a tribute to Jones's foundational insight—the Indo-European language family must have branched from a single trunk that sprouted many thousands of years ago, somewhere in the region of the Black Sea. By modern calculations that ancestral tongue (called *Proto Indo-European*, because it is strictly theoretical) would have existed around 4000–3000 BCE. It would have been the language of the Eurasian steppes at the time when steppe dwellers began to herd cattle and live in wagons, pioneering a nomadic herdsman's way of life. Because it was never written, Proto Indo-European can be reconstructed only indirectly, by identifying commonalities in languages that descend from it. Like a composite sketch drawn from the descriptions of various eyewitnesses, historical linguistics provides a rough likeness at best. Still, it tells us that the speakers of Proto Indo-European were patrilineal, sacrificed horses to sky gods, and used cannabis.

To trace this extremely ancient history, one speaks in millennia, as follows. In the third millennium, from 3000 to 2000 BCE, horse nomads of the steppes spread from the region north of the Black Sea far to the east, all the way to the Altai Mountains. The Altai Mountains partially interrupt the steppe, in Central Asia; beyond lies Mongolia. Central Asia has great relevance to our story because it seems to be the original homeland of the cannabis plant, where undomesticated varieties of it still grow along the road. If eastward-moving steppe nomads did not have cannabis already, they got it here.

In the second millennium, between 2000 and 1000 BCE, the steppes were fully "opened," acquiring their preeminent world-historical function as the migratory highway, trade crossroads, and strategic heart of Asia. Within a few hundred years of 1600 BCE, chariot technology, which apparently first arose on the edge of the steppes, spread to both ends of the east–west corridor, appearing in the Middle East and along China's northern frontier. At the same time, India saw the arrival of the chariot-driving, horse-sacrificing Vedic people. Before leaving the steppes, the Vedic people seem to have paused for a few centuries on the doorstep of Central Asia (the gap between the Aral Sea and the Himalayas), before descending into India with their Indo-European language, their herds of cattle, and their bhang drink. Although largely desert, this Central Asian doorstep had rich agricultural oases where Russian archeologists have unearthed what they believe to be temples that made and dispensed mind-altering drinks similar to soma or bhang. The evidence includes poppies, the pollen of prehistoric ephedra, and traces of cannabis. To find psychoactive drinks dispensed at a temple would be predictable, rather than surprising. Among the Vedic people, soma was drunk only during sacred rituals, and only by Brahmins, the priestly caste.

In the last millennium before the Common Era, between 1000 BCE and 1 CE, a new trick of Asia's mobile pastoralists made chariots outmoded. That innovation was learning to fight on horseback, and the crucial technologies were stirrups, which freed the hands from holding on, and the "composite bow" (composed of wood, bone, sinew, and glue), short enough to be easily handled in the saddle, powerful enough eventually to pierce armor. Stirrups, the composite bow, abundant mounts, and thousands of hours of practice made steppe warriors into horse archers like the mamluks whom we have already encountered in the medieval Muslim world. Horse archers could let fly ten to twenty arrows a minute, left- or right-handed, while galloping toward or away from (or in circles around) their enemies. Nothing so impressed anyone about them as their devastating effectiveness in warfare.

These steppe nomads of the period between 1000 BCE and 1 CE emerge vividly in a combination of archeological and literary evidence. The Eurasian steppe is treeless and dotted with thousands of easily visible mounds under which lie tombs from the last millennium BCE. Because these tomb-mounds are so obvious, most have been plundered over the centuries. Still, many have yielded helpful archeological information. A few have been "frozen tombs." These flooded soon after the burial and remained in solid permafrost until they were discovered and excavated by Russian archeologists in the twentieth century. Frozen tombs preserved the tattooed bodies of their occupants, clothing, weapons, the world's oldest "Persian" carpet, and surprising physical evidence of psychoactive cannabis use. We'll look at it in a moment.

A rare bit of literary evidence will help interpret the archaeology. It comes from the illustrious Greek historian Herodotus, who wrote in the mid-400s BCE. Herodotus visited the northern shore of the Black Sea and wrote at length about the steppe people. He called them Scythians, and they became the European archetype of frightful steppe "barbarians." (The ancient Greeks called most non-Greeks "barbarians.") Unlike later steppe people (Huns and Mongols, for example), Scythian horse archers were often blond and blue-eyed. Nazi myth-makers liked to imagine them as "Aryan" warrior forebears. Herodotus believed that among the Scythians were female warriors called Amazons, and archeologists have indeed found tombs of Scythian women buried with weapons. At one point, after describing the kind of lavish royal funeral in which scores of servants were executed and interred along with their king to accompany him to the underworld, Herodotus describes an act of self-purification practiced by surviving Scythian mourners after the tomb was sealed. The famous passage is often cited but rarely quoted in full, which is too bad:

> After the burial, those engaged in it have to purify themselves, which they do in the following way. First they soap and wash their heads. Then, to cleanse their bodies, they act as follows: they make a small structure by fixing in the ground three sticks inclined towards one another and stretching felt cloth around them as tightly as possible. Inside the structure a dish is placed upon the ground, and into it a number of red-hot stones, and then some cannabis seed.
>
> Cannabis, a plant that grows in Scythia, is very like flax, only much coarser and taller. Some grows wild; some is produced by cultivation. The Thracians make garments of cannabis fiber which closely resemble flaxen linen—so much so, indeed, that if a person has never seen cannabis he is sure to think the garments are of flax, and unless he is very experienced in such matters, he will not know of which material they are.
>
> The Scythians, as I said, take some of this cannabis seed, and, crawling under the felt coverings, throw it upon the red-hot stones, where it fills the enclosure with vapor as in a Greek steam bath, and the Scythians, delighted, shout for joy. The vapor replaces a water bath, for they never wash their bodies with water.

Herodotus often wrote from hearsay, his knowledge of Scythia was limited to one visit of a few months, and he was known to repeat a tall tale or two. So we need to consider, for starters, whether

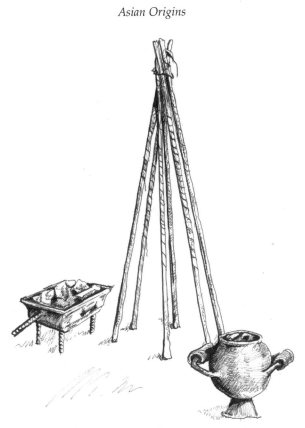

Scythian smoking set from a frozen tomb.

this account is credible at all. And what better corroboration than to find the very equipment that Herodotus described?

In the foothills of the Altai Mountains at a place called Pazyryk, early-twentieth-century Russian archeologist Sergei Rudenko found several frozen tombs containing two complete "smoking sets" (his term) exactly as described by Herodotus. Each was composed of (1) six wooden rods perforated at the top and tied together with a leather thong, (2) a leather or felt covering, and (3) a four-legged bronze brazier filled with crushed stone. The braziers' bronze handles were covered with bark so that they could be lifted when hot. Inside the braziers were cannabis seeds, some charred. Rudenko also found a small leather flask with unburned cannabis seeds attached to one of the wooden rods. The leather, felt, and wood had been preserved only because of the permafrost. Rudenko found the rods in every frozen tomb he opened. He believed that cannabis was being used not just after burials but as an everyday "narcotic" (his term), and by both women and men.

But were the Scythians really getting high in this way? Because cannabis seeds do not contain much (if any) THC, the Scythian technique would work psychoactively only if "smokers" were throwing the seeded, flowering tops of cannabis on the hot stones, rather than seeds alone. Moistened flowering tops would have emitted a mixture of smoke and steam as described by Herodotus. The ash, which was not found, would surely have washed away when the tombs flooded. There are other reports of this sort of "smoking" by related peoples who threw (unidentified) green plants on a fire to inhale the smoke. Similarly, temple incense in the ancient world as a whole involved inhaling the smoke of a smoldering censer in an enclosed space. A 2013 archaeological find in northern Pakistan suggests a similar practice in caves along the Kunar River in prehistoric times. On balance, though there are skeptics, archeologists today generally accept that the Scythians inhaled psychoactive cannabis smoke.

A close reading of Herodotus suggests that a psychoactive strain of cannabis was already separate from hemp. The people of the steppe had relatively little use for hemp fiber because, as with herding societies generally, their animals supplied abundant wool and leather to take the place of plant fibers. The frozen tombs contained hemp fiber only in the stitching of a few garments. In discussing the Scythian purification ritual, Herodotus digresses to compare cannabis to flax and tell how the Thracians (who live on the forested edge of the steppe) make fine linen of cannabis fiber. The Scythians did nothing comparable with the fiber, which is the reason for the digression. The Scythians apparently cultivated no hemp. And yet Herodotus specifies that while cannabis grew wild on the steppe, some was cultivated.

Herodotus also reveals that the Scythians weren't inhaling cannabis vapor merely for fun, even if it made them shout for joy. The purification ritual is described quite clearly as a cleansing bath, the only sort that Scythian men ever took. The bath involved spiritual, as well as physical, cleansing. Putting a deceased noble in a wagon for a farewell tour before burial, Scythian mourners traveled to the houses of friends and allies for banquets, during which the corpse was served food and drink along with the living. After socializing with the dead, though, the living needed to "purify themselves." Perhaps they encouraged the dead to sever their ties with the living by similar means. Upon opening the frozen tombs, the Russian archeologists found the tent-like structures standing with the braziers inside them. They had apparently been left smoldering when the tombs were closed.

For normal recreation, the Scythians didn't smoke, they drank. Perhaps, by this time, you saw that coming. Are you astonished to learn that the steppe nomads were enthusiastic drinkers of alcoholic beverages, be it wine, which they did not produce themselves, or fermented mare's milk, more or less their home brew? The Scythians were known *not* to mix their wine with water in the Greek fashion, and they had a taste for bingeing. Barbarians! "Drunk as a Scythian" was an ancient Greek expression, meaning very drunk, indeed. Successful warriors sometimes made ceremonial drinking cups from the skulls of their defeated enemies.

Scythian "smoking," in contrast, was spirit work, as was other Scythian drug use. Persian sources indicate that some groups of Scythians drank a psychoactive tea like Vedic soma. As a general pattern, fermented beverages were consumed mostly for enjoyment, but psychoactive beverages like Vedic soma were ritually prescribed and controlled. To judge by the Vedic hymns to soma, drinkers took its spirit into their bodies as a sort of worship, hoping for joy, wisdom, well-being, even immortality.

The early history of cannabis is still an unfolding story. Another frozen tomb along the steppe corridor was opened in 2008. This, too, was the burial of a mounted pastoralist, south of Pazyryk and the Altai Mountains, in the Gobi Desert. Today, that's western China. The tomb has been dated to around 700 BCE, more or less contemporary with the frozen tombs excavated in Russia. Along with a harp (one was also found at Pazyryk), bridles, and archery equipment, the Gobi tomb contained almost two pounds of cannabis leaves and female flowering tops in an excellent state of preservation, still green, in fact.

Specialists traveled from the United States to examine the cannabis and announced that it appeared to be a cultivated strain. Also, the male plants had evidently been culled. The tomb contained no smoking set, but the cannabis had been lightly pounded in a wooden bowl and placed in a leather basket, near the head of the mummy, possibly his equipment for steeping and straining the cannabis to make a psychoactive drink.

There will be more to say about forms of religion associated with early cannabis use in the last section of this chapter. For now, let us finish the story of how cannabis spread throughout Eurasia. Among the principal agents of this diffusion, apparently, were steppe people like the Scythians we have encountered in this section. Their military superiority made them all-conquering, and their migrations constituted the first great step in the global diffusion of cannabis.

THE SILK ROAD AND BEYOND

Once the horse archers of the steppe had gained a decisive military advantage over everyone around them, they went wherever they chose. Generally, that wasn't north, into the frozen coniferous forests of Siberia. It was east, west, and south, which is to say, China, Europe, and India. They carried cannabis with them, and their diverging paths created the great divide between *sativa* and *indica*. Observe.

The steppe is frigid, which made the south particularly appealing. But the steppe is bounded on the south by a series of barriers—mountains, deserts, inland seas—making it difficult to exit in a southerly direction. The most privileged place of north–south transit, historically, was the space between the Aral Sea and the Himalayas. There, thirsty travelers from the steppe could depend on rivers that flow down from the mountains to create fertile oases in the desert. We've been referring to this place as the doorstep of Central Asia, but now we'll be more precise, and call it the "Oxus" region, Oxus being the ancient name of its most important river, the Amu Darya.

The ancient people of this region, the Sogdians, spoke an Indo-European language and maintained close links to India and China. The Oxus region was on the Silk Road, the axis of land communication between the major early civilizations of Eurasia. The Sogdians preceded many of those civilizations, just as they preceded the silk trade itself, but the Oxus was already a crossroads by 2000 BCE. Sogdian dancing girls became famous in China for a whirling dance not unlike that of later dervishes. Not far away, Haydar supposedly "discovered" hashish when he saw a cannabis plant swaying on a quiet day. The Oxus, most likely, is where the cannabis plant was first cultivated to augment its potency as a drug. The Silk Road made it a perfect location.

Recall that a hot, dry climate encourages cannabis flowers to produce cannabinoids. The Altai region where cannabis still grows wild is much too northerly for the cultivation of high-potency cannabis. The more southerly Oxus region does possess such a climate, however, and so does another nearby region, the Taklamakan Desert, also on the Silk Road. The two pounds of cannabis recently discovered in a Gobi Desert tomb were probably cultivated on the edge of the Taklamakan. Ancient commercial hubs with a hot, dry climate would be ideal spots for the innovations that resulted in high-potency ganja and, much later, in modern hashish (charas), the concentrated resin, a product even better suited to long-distance trade.

Silk-route caravans that traversed the world's largest continent needed products that were rare and refined, imperishable and highly valued, neither heavy nor fragile—like silk itself. What better item than high-grade sin semilla? With the item traveled the know-how and, in a separate bag, the seeds. And where the trade most especially went, by all indications, was India. Persia, too, of course. But scorching and populous India became itself the greatest consumer and, eventually, producer of the drug. Perhaps sin semilla technique was created there, then spread to the Oxus region. That's possible, too. But the invention of charas certainly didn't occur in India. Silk Road origins have seemed more likely to me since the day I read, in the *Indian Hemp Drugs Commission Report*, that 1890s India imported its charas mostly from the Oxus region and the southern edge of the Taklamakan Desert.

Meanwhile, people were migrating east and west off the steppe, along more northerly latitudes, into China and Europe, too. There are some indications that wild cannabis had preceded them. Studies of prehistoric pollen indicate the possibility that cannabis had spread east and west to opposite ends of Eurasia well before the domestication of plants and animals. China and Europe would eventually become the world's main areas of cannabis cultivation, but their crops would remain strictly hemp, a matter of both cultivation and climate. No sort of cannabis plant could develop abundant cannabinoids, it seems, when planted on the shores of the Yellow River or the Baltic Sea.

The Chinese apparently adopted hemp from the steppe pastoralists who appeared on their northern border in the second millennium BCE. Traces of the nomads' arrival—the bones of horses—are unmistakable in the Lung-shan Neolithic farming culture that was then emerging on the alluvial plains of the Yellow River. Then, around 1200 BCE, in the Shang Dynasty, the first of China's long imperial history, there's even more unmistakable evidence of the steppe people's influence: a chariot burial. Archeologists have also recovered portions of hempen cloth from a Shang-period site in the far north. The horse archers of the northern border would play a constant and, occasionally, a leading role in Chinese history. The Great Wall was built and rebuilt over centuries to keep them out, but to no avail.

The Chinese were the first to cultivate cannabis on a large scale, and China's hemp crop has probably always been the world's largest. Some less-than-conclusive archeological finds even predate the arrival of the steppe dwellers. Impressions made by a woven textile on a still-wet pottery surface have been found at sites associated with Yang-shao Neolithic farming culture, the earliest of which there is any evidence in China. These finds could reach back as far as 4000 BCE, and the textile in question was probably hempen, but the imprints do not permit positive identification. In addition, there are several even older cordage imprints that also may have been made by cannabis, such as one on the island of Taiwan, from a period *preceding* the emergence of China's Yellow River civilization. Perhaps these are associated with the seafaring ancestors of the Polynesians, who are believed to have sailed into the Pacific from China's southern coast in Neolithic times. If these cordage and textile imprints are of cannabis, they represent the earliest sign of human usage.

In contrast to India, China possesses a wealth of written evidence. It shows that hemp was China's original fiber crop. *Ma*, the written Chinese character, or ideogram, that means "fiber," represents a couple of harvested cannabis plants hung up to dry. Ma continued to clothe the masses even after the upper classes took to wearing silk. Moreover, early texts indicate that cannabis seeds were a food source in ancient China, an unusual thing. Hempseed is quite nutritious and not bad tasting, but it doesn't keep well. Therefore, it was a seasonal, peasant food. Traditional Chinese histories, agricultural manuals, and Confucian rites—classic texts copied and recopied over millennia—are full of references to cannabis as both a fiber and a food crop. Eventually these texts were written on another great Chinese invention, paper, which was originally made of hemp fibers. (When Europeans copied papermaking from China, they too used hemp fibers at first.) The ancient Chinese made quite a science of hemp cultivation, prizing the female plant for its seed but preferring the male plant for its fiber. Ancient Chinese writing had six distinct characters for (1) cannabis in general, (2) male cannabis plants, (3) female cannabis plants, (4) male cannabis flowers, (5) cannabis seeds, and (6) cannabis "fruiting clusters."

There is some minimal indication of psychoactive cannabis in early Chinese history. *Ma* has figurative meanings suggesting psychoactive effects, for example. *Ma* (fiber) + *tsui* (drunkenness) form a compound meaning, generically, "mind-altering drug." It is also significant that the ancient Chinese had a specific word for cannabis "fruiting clusters," the seeded, flowering tops that the Scythians threw onto the hot rocks in their inhalation tents. A few medical texts mention psychoactive cannabis, and logically so, given China's ongoing contact with the Oxus and Taklamakan regions. The *Pen-Ts'ao Ching*, a pharmacopoeia written a mere two millennia ago, but preserving lore perhaps twice that old, says that the plant's fruiting clusters made one "see devils," but that, over time, they facilitated communication with spirits. Later, the famous physician T'ao Hung Ching wrote that the fruiting clusters of cannabis were no longer much prescribed, but that "sorcerers" combined them with ginseng "to reveal future events." Such prescriptions would have been administered, like many in Chinese medicine, as drinks.

In contrast, alcohol and other, unidentified psychoactive substances left robust substantiation of their presence in early Shang times. Shang emperors ruled over Bronze Age settlements in the valley of the Yellow River, where imperial China had its beginnings. Shang emperors exercised their rule partly by performing divination ceremonies. In fact, the oldest evidence of Chinese writing is etched onto "oracle bones," of which archeologists have discovered thousands. Acting as high-level shamans, Shang emperors posed questions to their ancestor spirits, and inscribed them on animal bones. The bones were then heated until they fractured, with the pattern of the fractures indicating answers from the spirit world. A fermented grog, possibly including fruiting clusters of cannabis, may have helped induce a trance in these divination ceremonies. The idea is speculative, however. As for ancient China's recreational drug, that was unquestionably alcohol. The greatest surviving artistic achievements of the Shang period are massive, elaborate bronze vessels that the nobility used as punch bowls for drinking parties.

Shamanic communication with the spirit world declined in China, beginning with the Confucian era, well over two thousand years ago, and the Confucian ethic, with its strong emphasis on duty, authority, hierarchy, and tradition, seems particularly inimical to the visionary, subversive affinities of cannabis drugs. China never developed a major tradition of drug-using religious ascetics like Sannyasins or dervishes. In contrast, many quite respectable Chinese did become habitual consumers of opium when it was introduced by Arab traders in the Common Era, perhaps because opium's effects were more suitable to their needs. Drowsy opium induces contentment rather than dissidence, one could say. That idea, at any rate, has been proposed by a Chinese scholar, who also says that sometimes, in centuries past, the older generation of prosperous families *wanted* to see the younger generation use opium because its sedative effects would keep them out of trouble. He adds that in the early twentieth century, the Uyghurs, an ethnic minority group who live in western China, grew cannabis for exportation to India and also consumed it themselves, while their ethnic Chinese neighbors refused to touch the stuff. Even today, cannabis drugs have virtually no presence on China's national scene. Without published statistics, it's hard to say anything more precise. Meanwhile, China grows about 40 percent of the world's hemp.

Now let's rewind our chronology to trace the much slower emergence of the world's other great hemp crop, that of northern Europe. For centuries, Europeans' main supplement for local hemp supplies came from the shores of the Baltic Sea. Europe's story can be more quickly summarized than China's, because hemp has played a smaller role in European life.

Historical linguists have reconstructed the expansion of the Indo-European language family as Celtic, Germanic, and Slavic tongues swept slowly west from the steppe across northern Europe. That hemp-bearing westward flow occurred in successive waves, beginning in the third millennium BCE, leaving behind it distinctive types of pottery from Russia to Poland to France. One type is called "corded ware" because it is decorated by the marks of a twisted cord that was pressed into the wet clay. Andrew Sherratt, a leading archeologist of Neolithic Europe, suggested that the cord impressions are consistent with twisted hemp rope, and that, because corded ware is often made in the size and shape of drinking cups, it may have contained a psychoactive cannabis drink. However, fiber and drug crops don't usually go together, as we know, and the impressions cannot be conclusively identified anyway.

In Europe, other fibers competed more successfully with hemp. Europe's original fiber plant was flax, and Europe also possessed more wool and fur than China. Because of its extremely long fibers, though, hemp made the best cordage of any European plant, so early Europeans kept a bit on hand for rope. The Celts supplied hemp fiber or cordage to the Romans, who used it to rig their ships. By the Viking period, Scandinavians cultivated hemp for the same purpose. Later, as global exploration got under way, Europe's major seafaring nations all worked to ramp up their own hemp production. In sum, it was the great expansion of European seaborne trade and naval competition that made hemp an important European crop.

As for cannabis drugs, European hemp produced none. Europe was the most northerly destination of the cannabis plant's global diffusion, a circumstance *not* conducive to cannabinoids. Unlike the Chinese, Europeans lost touch with Central Asia during the centuries when the southern strain was being developed as a drug crop. Knowledge of the plant's drug potential, and how to cultivate it, seems not to have reached Western Europe before the nineteenth century. Overall, compelling evidence of psychoactive cannabis is totally absent from Europe until around 1800, when French soldiers returned with hashish from Napoleon's failed Egyptian expedition.

A few titillating clues do exist. A "pipe cup" found in Bucharest suggests at least the possibility of Scythian-style inhalation there in the third century BCE. Then there's the Oseberg ship burial in Norway, from a thousand years later, around 850 CE. It contained a single hempseed in a leather pouch buried with a woman who may have been a pagan priestess. Also, there's a 1562 recipe for an Italian witches' brew that supposedly calls for female cannabis flowers. And cannabis resin was reportedly found in a pipe excavated from the vicinity of Shakespeare's house in Stratford, England. These clues are thought-provoking, certainly, but they are outliers. An overwhelming mass of negative evidence (basically, *everything* else known about European history) indicates *no* significant use of psychoactive cannabis, ever, in traditional European society. At most, the unexplained clues above indicate the possibility of an awareness, shared by very few Europeans (the world's most prodigious consumers of ethanol), that cannabis might possess psychoactive properties, or perhaps, had once possessed them.

It *is* interesting, though, that several of these clues point in a familiar direction. Who may have known something, anything at all, about the potentially psychoactive powers of cannabis in historic Europe? A pagan priestess or a witch, two people outside

of Europe's dominant religion. The priestess of the Oseberg ship burial was pre-Christian and certainly had access to religious lore of a kind that we can loosely call "shamanic." The witches of early modern Europe, too, may have preserved some access to that lore—whatever remained of Europe's ancient shamanic religions having become witchcraft in Christian eyes. Shamanism is the last, which is to say, the *earliest* horizon in our backward survey of the global history of marijuana. The earliest regular users of cannabis drugs were almost certainly shamans. It is time we gave shamanism a closer look.

THE EARLIEST HORIZON

Okay, so here's the Anthropology 101 version.

Shamans are religious specialists characteristic of hunter-gatherer, also called foraging, societies. Before eleven or twelve thousand years ago more or less all humans were foragers. Basic elements of shamanic practice have been cataloged and studied by travelers and anthropologists over the last two centuries. They exhibit an unmistakable family resemblance around the world from the indigenous inhabitants of northern Europe and Asia, especially Siberia, to the native people of the Americas, from Alaska right down to Tierra del Fuego. To have spread so widely, this cultural pattern must have crossed from Asia to the Americas during the last ice age, before the domestication of plants and animals. Therefore, an understanding of shamanism may help us imagine spiritual life from the time before humans lived in villages or grew food, but instead, foraged in family groups, frequently on the move. That early spiritual life was almost certainly the context within which we discovered the psychoactive properties of cannabis.

In the last half-century, various scholars have identified what they believe to be traces of shamanism in prehistoric art. The most persuasive single example is a twelve-thousand-year-old painting of a half-man, half-beast (or possibly, a man wearing an owl mask, stag horns, a lion's skin, and a horse's tail) discovered deep in a French cavern, the famous "dancing sorcerer." Another Paleolithic

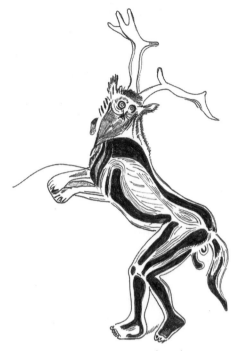

Dancing Sorcerer, apparently a shaman.

cave painting shows a stick figure, apparently wearing a bird mask, prostrate on the ground as if in a trance (he has an erection), a bird-headed staff (such as shamans still use) lying beside him. Archeologists working on more recent Neolithic sites have identified tomb decorations they believe to be shamanic in Ireland and other parts of Europe's Celtic fringe. These decorations are not paintings of human and animal figures, but rather geometric patterns engraved into the surface of the rock. Comparing them with drawings by contemporary shamans, these archeologists argue that the patterns in Neolithic tombs represent "entoptic phenomena," abstract visual patterns that shamans see in trance visions. This "psychedelic" art flanks entrance tunnels to the tombs, perhaps symbolizing access to the underworld.

Altered states of consciousness are basic to shamanism. Shamans do their work in a state of trance, sometimes lying apparently unconscious and later reporting visions, other times, depending on the traditions that are infinitely variable in their details, miming actions and speaking in voices to an audience that participates in the ceremony. Most shamanic trances are not drug-induced, but many are. Drugs used by shamans to induce a trance are termed *entheogens*, a word meaning that they "awaken the divine within." All psychoactive drugs, including alcohol and tobacco, have been employed as entheogens. Spanish drug scholar Antonio Escohotado divides various substances into "possession" drugs that are oblivion-producing sedatives (alcohol, opium) and "tripping" drugs that produce hallucinations recalled afterward, by the tripper, in vivid detail. The most frequently used entheogens are hallucinogens, such as peyote cactus, psilocybin mushrooms, *Amanita muscaria* mushrooms, or ayahuasca vines. Cannabis is less hallucinogenic than these drugs, but it is, nonetheless, one of world's most widespread entheogens.

Working in a state of altered consciousness distinguishes shamans from other "technicians of the sacred," like sorcerers or priests, who often exist alongside shamans. The shaman's function is specific and limited. Shamanic trances enable interaction with the spirit world. In a trance, the shaman's spirit can leave his body and fly to the spirit realm above the normal plane of human existence, or tunnel to the spirit realm below it. A typical shamanic cosmology consists of a multitiered universe with several levels above and below ground, often joined by a "world tree" whose branches hold up the sky and whose roots give access to the underworld. Shamans are often employed to guide the spirits of the dead to their subterranean destination. They know the route, so to speak. Recall, in this connection, those psychedelic entrances to Neolithic tombs, and consider that the Paleolithic cave paintings were normally quite deep underground. Such paintings could never be viewed under normal circumstances and were clearly magical in intent.

Shamans can consult with the omniscient spirits, who are often ancestors, in order to know what the future will bring and, sometimes, to assure good fortune. (This is what the Shang emperors were apparently doing.) Moreover, their interaction with spirits allows shamans to heal the sick. People call a shaman when they attribute illness to the intrusion of a malignant spirit or to a weakening of the patient's own spirit.

Hunter-gatherers are generally animists who envision a world alive with spirits, the spirits of people, living and dead, of course, but also the spirits of animals. Animal spirits are crucial for hunters, naturally—as prey, as rival predators whom hunters honor and emulate, as lead players in the hunters' cast of mythic characters. The shaman's chief allied spirits usually appear as animals. Like flying, changing into an animal is a frequent scenario of shamanic trance. Animal masks and disguises, as well as animal teeth, bones, and feathers are standard shamanic attire. In a trance, shamans may don the attire to "become" the animal. Shamans know the spirits of places, such as mountains and rivers, and also of plants. Shamans who consume an entheogenic plant are taking its spirit into their bodies. They often speak directly to the plant spirit and entreat its aid, as do the Vedic hymns to soma.

An entheogen is never "recreational." The shaman's spiritual work is just that, work. It is often ecstatic—which is to say, involving an "out-of-body" experience—but it has nothing to do with euphoria. A man or woman receives the calling to become a shaman. The aspirant then undergoes a period of apprenticeship, learning spirit lore from a master. Often, a crucial part of this training is the collection, preparation, and ritual consumption of entheogens. Shamanic knowledge of entheogens is usually secret. They are, by definition, not for everyone, at least most of the time. Some shamans supervise initiation rituals by which boys and girls become adult members of hunter-gatherer societies, and the ritual is often an ordeal during which the initiates consume entheogens. Usually, however, the entheogens are for the shaman alone. They are a tool of the trade.

A shaman uses entheogens to see what others can't. Consider the difference between shamans and priests, who are characteristic of later, larger, agricultural societies in global history. Priests are above all keepers of detailed, arcane knowledge, inscribed in sacred texts or memorized verbatim. When priests enact the rituals as prescribed, they deploy a spiritual power that inheres in the rituals themselves. The efficacy of the Catholic Mass, for example, depends not at all on the personal qualities of the priest who officiates. The priest's script, so to speak, is everything, his personal ability, nothing. In contrast, personal ability is crucial for a shaman, whose arcane knowledge consists mostly in a set of techniques enabling him to operate within the spirit world. Shamans' interventions may be somewhat scripted, but they necessarily involve improvisation. In sum, priests may sense a spiritual presence, but their work does not depend on it, while shamans *must* sense a spiritual presence and interact with it. Their success depends largely on imagination and creativity.

The world's best-known shaman ever is probably the one depicted by Carlos Castañeda in *The Teachings of Don Juan: A Yaqui Way of Knowledge* (1968), a published version of the author's doctoral dissertation in anthropology. The book made a stir and spawned best-selling sequels. The field research has been challenged, but the representation of shamanic training is highly informed and provides an excellent illustration. Don Juan, an ordinary looking, elderly Mexican of indigenous descent, is a man of few words. He explains virtually nothing about the spirit world. Instead, he gives Castañeda precise instructions on how to prepare and ingest three entheogens—peyote, datura, and psilocybin mushrooms—each of which is understood as a spirit and, potentially, an "ally." To make friends with a potential ally, the author is instructed to dance in front of the plant on successive days. Eventually, he ingests the entheogens one by one, on separate occasions, to audition with their spirits, so to speak. Different shamans find different allies, a matter of personal affinities. Castañeda's experiences vary from baffling to terrifying, the furthest thing imaginable from "recreational." The teachings of Don Juan are, in essence, a set of supervised, drug-induced trances, training for a would-be visionary. The spiritual insights acquired by the apprentice come not from the teacher's words but from direct, personal experience.

In sum, entheogens are used as part of a spiritual quest, and cannabis is among the world's most frequent entheogens. Physical evidence of cannabis drugs before around 700 BCE is limited and questionable, but whenever and however it took place, the first regular use of cannabis to alter consciousness probably occurred in a shamanic context. That knowledge creates a meaningful chronological starting place for the narrative of marijuana's global history, and consequently, a fitting conclusion for our backward exploration of it.

6

✳

Epiphanies

Histories of cannabis commonly invoke its great antiquity as a domesticated plant, and its antiquity cannot be doubted. Just as commonly, though, one finds a mistaken impression of how the plant was being used during several millennia. Psychoactive cannabis figures in global history mostly as an entheogen, employed less for its euphoriant properties than for its visionary epiphanies.

The widespread use of marijuana as a recreational drug is rare and recent in world history. To be sure, the use of cannabis drugs is at least three thousand years old, and probably older. During most of that time, however, it has belonged especially to shamans and, then, to mystical ascetics who hungered for direct, personal access to divinity. Hindu and Muslim civilizations are the two main contexts in which cannabis drugs appear during the last millennium, and ascetic holy men were their most typical users in each case. Recreational use, which draws on marijuana's euphoriant qualities rather than its hallucinogenic qualities, has been strikingly less important in global history. The seasonal bhang-drinking tradition of northern India aside, there is no evidence that cannabis has replaced alcohol as the general recreational euphoriant in any major world society, ever.

Where cannabis *has* been used recreationally, it has been as a poor man's drug, a more affordable substitute for ethanol, often adopted by people who are socially and ethnically marginalized. That was true, apparently, south of the Congo River, in the wake of the slave trade, and true also throughout Latin America, which has had, overall, less experience with psychoactive cannabis than has the United States. Migrating workers carried marijuana around the Western Hemisphere in the late nineteenth and early twentieth centuries. In the United States, the 1960s counterculture changed the social profile of marijuana as millions of middle-class young people adopted it, and the prestige of the U.S. example inspired international imitation. Today's high prices appear all the more unprecedented when one thinks that, consistently for the previous several thousand years until only a few decades ago, the main users of cannabis drugs have been the poor, most notably wandering holy men who lived by begging.

The privileged place of alcohol turns out to be absolutely standard in global history. No other single discovery of this investigation impressed me more. In global perspective, cannabis and alcoholic beverages have hugely asymmetrical profiles. Ethanol is *food*, full of calories, whether we want them or not. It is consumed avidly by birds that find it in fermented berries. Fermentation is a natural food preservative. Myriad forms of wine and beer are produced from the earliest domesticated plants and have been a regular part of the human diet around the world since the invention of agriculture. The volume of alcohol consumption has varied radically from place to place. Anyone short on food is unlikely to make much ethanol. Various religious strictures have limited it. However, most human societies have used alcohol to some degree. Europe has made and consumed ethanol with special intensity, and European colonialism has intensified consumption in the rest of the world. If drug traffic is the transport and sale of mind-altering substances, then the most trafficked drug in history has always been ethanol.

By comparison, marijuana is a recreational Johnny-come-lately whose adoption by middle-class people made it the world's most used illegal drug only in the late twentieth century. The United States (with an annual prevalence around 13 percent) is now the world capital of marijuana cultivation and use, followed by other developed countries. Various European countries (Spain, Portugal) have recently liberalized their drug laws, others (Sweden, France, the UK) have not, and some (the Netherlands) have made laws more restrictive. The famous hashish cafés of Amsterdam have closed their doors to tourists. Meanwhile, Latin American countries are beginning to legalize or decriminalize marijuana in self-defense against the criminal traffic and its attendant mayhem, but only Jamaica consumes at U.S. levels. Most parts of the world where marijuana (in hashish and other forms) has been consumed for many centuries now use less. South Asia consumes at only a fraction of U.S. levels, even though marijuana continues to play a role in religious observance in several countries, including India. Estimates for Africa vary, but even the high guesses do not exceed U.S. levels. In Thailand, once famous for its marijuana, stylish young people have switched to methamphetamine. In burgeoning China, where cannabis was first intensively cultivated, marijuana use is close to unknown. The highlight of a recent marijuana-oriented tour of the world outside of North America and Western Europe was Australia, where the small New South Wales town of Nimbin hosts an annual "Mardi Grass" festival.

Cannabis drugs have never been for everybody. Instead, they have consistently been used by people seeking meditative insights, a stimulus to creativity, direct access to the spirit world, or the experience of transcending earthly cares to enter a mystical union with God and the cosmos. This last phenomenon, called the "unitive experience," is among the most esteemed and ecstatic in the world. This what those hashish-eating Sufis and ganja-smoking Sannyasins were after, an experience prized by our greatest prophets and religious teachers, typically a pivotal moment in any life. Yet those who seek it are a small minority in any society.

How hallucinogenic drugs like marijuana might contribute to spiritual insights remains a mystery. Very little scientific study of them has been done since the 1960s. That study has recommenced, however, and just as was true in the 1960s, subjects exposed to powerful psychedelic drugs in controlled trials still report profound experiences with a lasting effect. Moreover, new tools are providing a different view of the phenomenon. Digital imaging that traces blood flow in the brain, for example, shows that hallucinogens (psilocybin, at least) reduce activity in parts of the brain that neuroscientists term "the default-mode network." Intriguingly, some believe the default-mode network to be the physical, neurological home of the self or ego. Its reduced activity would therefore imply diminished feelings of self or ego, which precisely describes the unitive experience.

Allen Ginsberg would certainly not be surprised to learn, had he lived to see this new focus of neuroscience, that the brains of people on psychedelic drugs operate less in something called "default mode." Suppression of default mode sounds very much like his description of the way marijuana affected his thinking. Many other writers, musicians, artists, and generally creative people believe that marijuana stimulates their creativity in a similar manner, contributing to what nonartists might call "thinking outside the box." The brain's default-mode network has also been compared to an orchestra conductor. Suppress the brain's conductor, it seems, and you unleash powers of improvisation and . . . start to get jazz. This kind of creativity, rather than a concerted effort, is a release. The power to create seems to come out of nowhere and is often believed to be a spiritual gift. "Inhaling a divine breath" is the ancient, root meaning of *inspiration*, the gift of the muse. Inspired ideas seem to appear all at once, fully formed in consciousness, like epiphanies.

And there's the rub. Not everyone relishes creative and philosophical epiphanies. They are often lonely experiences, and unshared epiphanies can be disconcerting for all concerned. Religious epiphanies may be taken for divine revelations, and the major world religions, mainly based on past revelations recorded in scripture, look askance on claims of divine revelation in the present. Christianity and Islam, with their emphasis on liturgical authority, mostly reject entheogens. From a mainstream Christian or Muslim perspective, the time for prophetic visions is over. Entheogens somehow represent "the competition," sometimes the devil. In the United States today this critique is not made in religious terms and is, perhaps, not even self-conscious. Moreover, marijuana's euphoriant qualities, the basis of its recreational appeal, worry many religious people, because the euphoria seems unearned and, therefore, immoral. The objection that medical marijuana users will feel better partly because they are high is essentially moralistic. It accompanies the worry that marijuana users are disrespecting traditional models. All these feelings have deep historical roots.

Those who worry about marijuana need not be so fearful, however. Marijuana is unlikely to replace, or even rival, alcohol as our recreational drug of choice. It is not for everybody. For most people, its euphoriant effect is less than alcohol's. It is most likely to be used by the poor, by the marginal, by the chronically ill, by the artistically and philosophically and spiritually inclined, by seekers after the meaning of life, and by social and religious nonconformists of various stripes. That, at least, is the picture that emerges from this short global history. Marijuana, it seems, is a mind-expanding drug after all.

Glossary

Cannabis has had many forms in global history. Therefore this book requires many specific historical names, but it employs *marijuana* as the most general term.

bhang—Indian name for cannabis plant and a traditional, mildly psychoactive drink

bud—fully mature, resin-laden flowers of the female plant

cannabis—Indo-European genus name covering all forms of the plant, first recorded by Herodotus

   Cannabis sativa—scientific name given by Linnaeus to a domestic Swedish specimen (1753)

   Cannabis indica—scientific name given by Lamarck to an Indian specimen (1783)

   Cannabis ruderalis—scientific name given by Janischewski to a Central Asian specimen (1924)

   cannabinoids—molecules peculiar to resin of female cannabis flowers

   endocannabinoids—human hormones resembling cannabinoids

   endocannabinoid system—human physiological system regulated by cannabinoids and endocannabinoids

charas—Indian name of concentrated resin, similar to modern hashish

dagga—cannabis smoked in early South Africa

diamba—main Brazilian term for the drug in the early 1900s, an African word

fumo de Angola—roughly, Angola tobacco (Brazil, ca. 1900)

fumo de caboclo—roughly, Indian tobacco (Brazil, ca. 1900)

ganja—Indian term, imported to Jamaica in the 1800s, for *sin semilla*

"the green one"—medieval Arabic slang for hashish, contrasts with "the red one" (wine)

grifo—ca. 1920 Mexican slang for marijuana or marijuana cigarette

hashish—in medieval Arabic, equivalent of **ganja**; today, concentrated resin rich in cannabinoids, equivalent of **charas**

> **hashishi** (singular), **hashishiyya** or **hashishin** (plural)—medieval Arabic for "hashish eater(s)," a common slur, rendered "ashishin" by Marco Polo

hemp—*Cannabis sativa* that is **not** marijuana and is lacking in cannabinoids

maconha—principal name of Brazilian marijuana today

marijuana—psychoactive cannabis originating in Mexico

> **medical marijuana**—modern *sin semilla*, sold at dispensaries, often an *indica-sativa* hybrid
>
> **recreational marijuana**—same as the above, different application
>
> **marihuana**—original Spanish-language form of the word
>
> **María Juana**—slang verbal "disguise" for marijuana

marimba—Colombian term for *Cannabis indica*, imported into—then exported from—Colombia's Caribbean coast

pipiltzintzintlis—apparently, an Indigenous Mexican word applied to psychoactive cannabis in the 1700s

reefer (probably from **grifo**)—mid-1900s United States, originally African American

riamba—Central African word for psychoactive cannabis, apparently derived from **bhang**

> **Beni Riamba Brotherhood**—tribal society that attempted to settle conflicts by smoking **riamba**

Rosa María—in 1800s Mexico, a verbal disguise for marijuana

sin semilla—fully mature buds, never pollinated, for maximum drug potency; from Spanish, "without seeds"

Sources and Asides

As I've observed often in the preceding pages, the sources for a global history of marijuana are limited. This appendix offers notes on the most interesting and important ones available in English. It also includes asides on a few topics that may be of interest.

GETTING HIGH

I recommend several general histories of marijuana that provide an abundance of detail, especially regarding recent developments in the United States: Martin A. Lee, *Smoke Signals: A Social History of Marijuana—Medical, Recreational, and Scientific* (New York: Scribner, 2012); and Martin Booth, *Cannabis: A History* (New York: St. Martin's, 2003), which also covers the United Kingdom. Chris Duvall concentrates more on the global picture in *Cannabis* (London: Reaktion, 2015).

AMERICAN CENTURY

The last century of the story is by far the best known, and my telling of it is conventional. The indispensable study for the early twentieth-century is Richard J. Bonnie and Charles H. Whitebread,

The Marihuana Conviction: A History of Marijuana Prohibition in the United States (New York: Lindesmith Center, 1999). Those interested in jazz vipers should take a look at the memoir of Milton Mezzrow and Bernard Wolfe, *Really the Blues* (New York: Random House, 1946).

Some readers may have heard the argument that the 1937 Marihuana Tax Act resulted from a conspiracy joining Hearst interests (timber) and DuPont interests (synthetic fiber products) to outlaw competition from hemp. The case is plausible, but strictly circumstantial. It derives from an extraordinary book by Jack Herer, a leading spirit of the pro-hemp movement that began in the 1990s. Herer's self-published *The Emperor Wears No Clothes* (10th ed., 1995) is a remarkable phenomenon worthy of a look by any aficionado. Much of the book is a mass of photocopied primary sources, some almost in microform.

The La Guardia Report was published as Mayor's Committee on Marihuana, *The Marihuana Problem in the City of New York* (New York: Jacques Cattell, 1944).

ATLANTIC WORLD

David T. Courtwright provides a vigorous overview of the commercial globalization of drugs, encompassing not only distilled spirits but also tea, coffee, tobacco, and opium. Courtwright's economically driven model has less to say about marijuana, which did not become a commodity in international trade until much more recently. Still, Courtwright's concise and wide-ranging *Forces of Habit: Drugs and the Making of the Modern World* (Cambridge, MA: Harvard University Press, 2001) provides an ideal overview for readers interested in the global history of drugs.

Marijuana's early history in Latin America has long been the least understood portion of its global itinerary. Isaac Campos, *Home Grown: Marijuana and the Origin of Mexico's War on Drugs* (Chapel Hill: University of North Carolina Press, 2012) has begun to change that. Campos is my main source on Mexico, and I consider his book to be the best recent academic monograph on any aspect of marijuana history. Also de rigueur is the classic collection edited by Vera Rubin, *Cannabis and Culture* (The Hague: Mouton, 1975), with a number of chapters on Latin America. Though not in English, the essential source for Brazil is the compendium published as Ministério da Saúde, *Maconha: Coletânea de trabalhos brasileiros* (Rio de Janeiro: Serviço Nacional de Educação Sanitária, 1958). Finally, two studies of Colombia deserve mention: Lina Britto Londoño, "Contrabandistas, marimberos, y parranderos: Breve historia oral de la bonanza de la marihuana en la Guajira, 1970's," MA thesis, Department of Anthropology, Universidad de la Cordillera, La Paz, Bolivia, 2009; and Eduardo Sáenz Rovner, "La Prehistoria de la marihuana en Colombia: Consumo y cultivos entre los años 30 y 60," *Cuadernos de Economía* 26, no. 47 (2007): 205–22.

On Africa, see Chris Duvall, *Cannabis*, cited above, and Brian M. Du Toit, *Cannabis in Africa: A Survey of Its Distribution in Africa and a Study of Cannabis Use and Users in Multi-Ethnic South Africa* (Rotterdam: A. A. Balkema, 1980). The intriguing source on the Beni Riamba Brotherhood is Hermann von Wissman, *My Second Journey through Equatorial Africa from the Congo to the Zambesi, in the Years 1886 and 1887* (London: Chatto & Windus, 1891).

MEDIEVAL HASHISH

Though difficult to absorb, abundant evidence from medieval manuscript sources in Arabic is marshaled authoritatively by the work of the distinguished Yale professor Franz Rosenthal, *The Herb: Hashish versus Medieval Muslim Society* (Leiden: E. J. Brill, 1971). This chapter is based primarily on that evidence along with an overall understanding of the medieval Muslim world. Another study crucial to my account is Ahmet T. Karamustafa, *God's Unruly Friends: Dervish Groups in the Islamic Later Middle Period* (Salt Lake City: University of Utah Press, 1994). Aficionados will also find much to savor in Hakim Bey and Abel Zug, *Orgies of the Hemp Eaters: Cuisine, Slang, Literature, & Ritual of Cannabis Culture* (New York: Autonomedia, 2004), a fabulous compendium of excerpts, essays, annotated bibliography, and primary sources on cannabis history in South Asia and the Muslim World. Passing references to hashish occur frequently in *One Thousand and One Nights,* but the drug is more or less central to three stories in particular: "The Tale of the Hashish Eater," "The Tale of the Two Hashish Eaters," and "The Tale of the Second Captain of Police." A variety of other tales have been collected by Andrew C. Kimmens, *Hashish Tales* (New York: Morrow, 1975).

See Booth, *Cannabis,* for a much fuller discussion of hashish experimenters in nineteenth-century Europe and the United States, including (on page 86) the quotation from Théophile Gautier, the creator of the Parisian Hashish Eaters Club. The writings of nineteenth-century European and U.S. experimenters make interesting reading without contributing much to the global history of marijuana. Fitz Hugh Ludlow's account has been reprinted as *The Hasheesh Eater: Being Passages from the Life of a Pythagorean* (New Brunswick, NJ: Rutgers University Press, 2006).

The history of modern hashish, the concentrated resin, is not covered by the present book, except for speculations in chapter 5 about its possible origins along the Silk Road. Its major exporters have been Lebanon, Morocco, Afghanistan, and Nepal. Egypt has been an important consuming country. Also not covered here is Moroccan *kif,* which is a mixture of chopped cannabis and tobacco. See Laurence Cherniak, *The Great Books of Hashish* (Berkeley, CA: And/Or Press, 1979).

ASIAN ORIGINS

The indispensable primary source for India has been reprinted as *Report of the Indian Hemp Drugs Commission, 1893–1894* (Silver Spring, MD: Jefferson, 1969), which provides the findings in one volume. An excellent account of the use of ganja by Indian sadhus (sannyasins) appears in Patricia Morningstar, "Thandai and Chilam: Traditional Hindu Beliefs about the Proper Uses of Cannabis," *Journal of Psychoactive Drugs* 17, no. 3 (1985): 141–65, reprinted in Bey and Zug, *Orgies.* Also see Khwaja A. Hasan, "Social Aspects of Cannabis Use in India," in Rubin, *Cannabis and Culture,* 235–45.

Soma, the ritual drink of the Vedic priestly caste, was basically a tea made of plants (especially one called soma) that were pulverized, steeped, and strained, as for the bhang drink. The soma plant itself has not been positively identified. In addition, "owing to the difficulty of obtaining the actual soma plant, several substitutes were used," and there were at least five possible admixtures that cannot be positively identified, either. The bhang plant was recognized as belonging to the "family" of soma and may have figured occasionally as one of its active ingredients. See Parati Ghosal, *Lifestyle of the Vedic People* (New Delhi: DKPrintworld, 2006).

The early prehistory of marijuana is still emerging and must be pieced together from scattered sources. See Duvall, *Cannabis*. The Herodotus quotation is from the classic 1910 *History of Herodotus*, translated by George Rawlinson, with a few modifications for the sake of clarity. (Rawlinson translated the word *cannabis* as "hemp," for example.) Duvall doubts that the famous account by Herodotus involved psychoactive cannabis, but the archeologist who unearthed the equipment described by the Greek historian had no doubts in the matter. See Sergei I. Rudenko, *Frozen Tombs of Siberia: The Pazyryk Burials of Iron Age Horsemen* (London: J. M. Dent and Sons, 1970; first published in Russian, 1953). The leading late-twentieth-century archeologist of prehistoric drug use agreed with Rudenko. See Andrew Sherratt, "Sacred and Profane Substances: The Ritual Use of Narcotics in Later Neolithic Europe," in *Economy and Society in Prehistoric Europe: Changing Perspectives* (Princeton, NJ: Princeton University Press, 1997), 403–30. David Lewis-Williams and David Pearce explore the prehistory of religion in *Inside the Neolithic Mind: Consciousness, Cosmos, and the Realm of the Gods* (London: Thames and Hudson, 2005).

EPIPHANIES

The long-term perspective, by which pagan "visionary drugs" become associated with witchcraft and the devil, is traced by Antonio Escohotado in *A Brief History of Drugs: From the Stone Age to the Stoned Age* (Rochester, VT: Park Street, 1999). Readers of Spanish should prefer Escohotado's three-volume original version, *Historia general de las drogas* (Madrid: Alianza Editorial, 1989), which contains many more examples.

Index

About the Author

John Charles Chasteen is a North Carolina writer, translator of Spanish and Portuguese, and, for twenty-five years, professor of history at UNC Chapel Hill, where he was born (on campus) in 1955. *Born in Blood and Fire*, his concise overview of Latin American history, is among the most read in the English language. Chasteen's abiding scholarly interest has been the emotional roots of nation and nationalism in nineteenth-century Latin America. His books on the topic include *Heroes on Horseback: A Life and Times of the Last Gaucho Caudillos* (1995), *National Rhythms, African Roots: A Deep History of Latin American Popular Dance* (2004), and *Americanos: Latin America's Struggle for Independence* (2008). Chasteen is also an award-winning editor and translator of Latin American fiction and nonfiction, most recently *The Alienist and Other Stories of Nineteenth-Century Brazil* (2012), by the Brazilian literary master Joaquim Machado de Assis, and *The Gaucho Juan Moreira* (2014), the classic Argentine "true crime" saga, by Eduardo Gutiérrez. He has a bilingual screenplay adaptation of W. H. Hudson's *The Purple Land*, if anyone knows a producer. He lives with his wife, Carmen, in the countryside near Chapel Hill.